Cutaneous Melanoma

Edited by Paweł Pietkiewicz

Published in London, United Kingdom

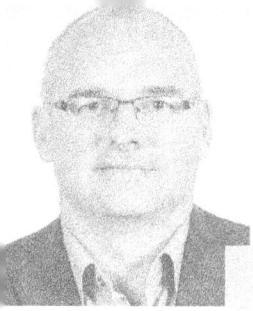
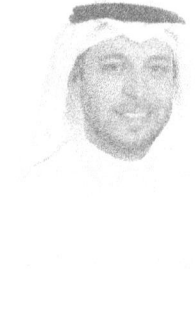
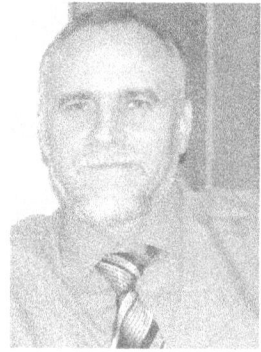
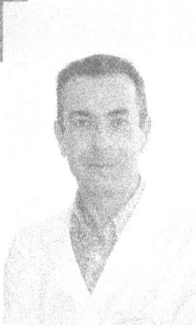
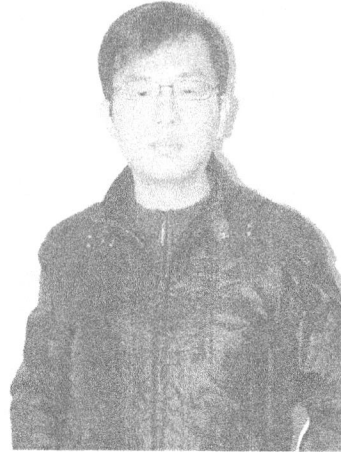
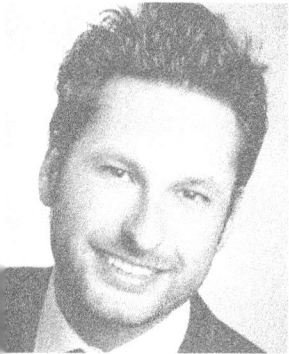
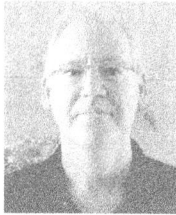

IntechOpen

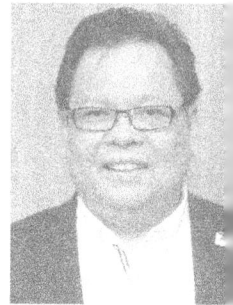
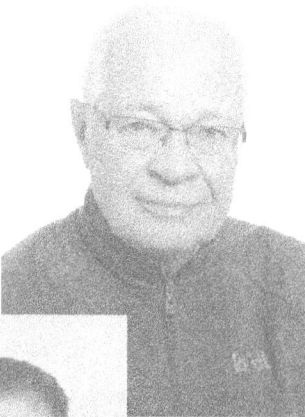
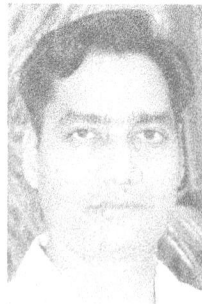
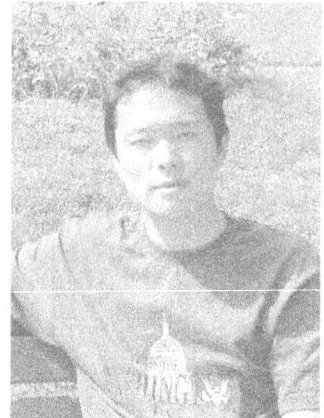
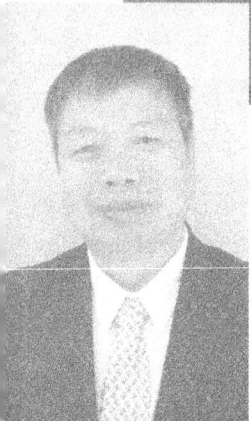
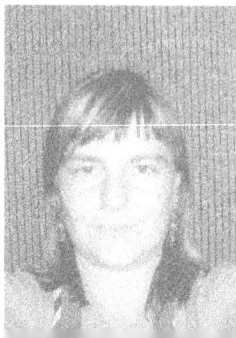

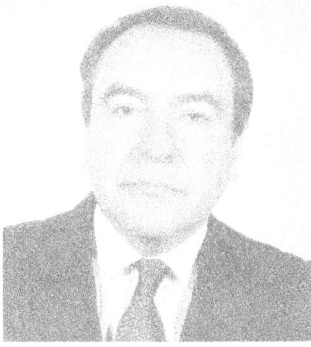

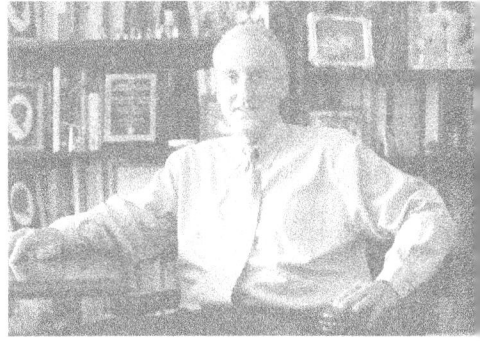

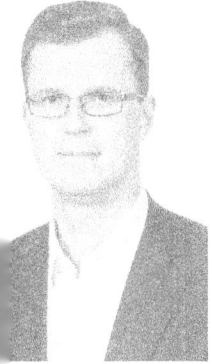

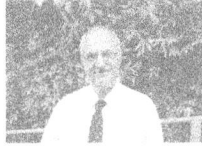

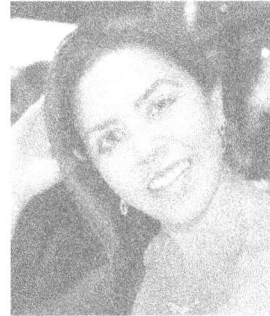

Supporting open minds since 2005

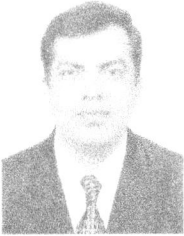

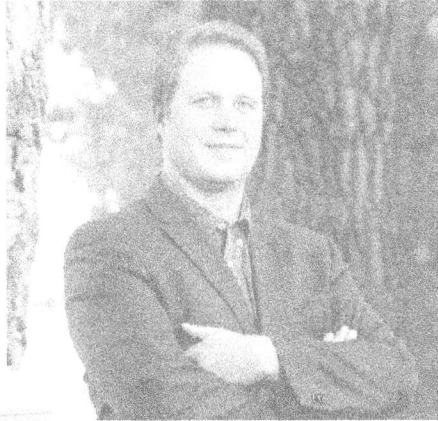

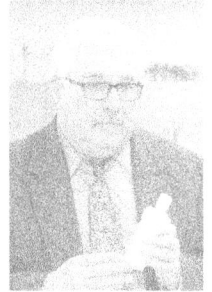

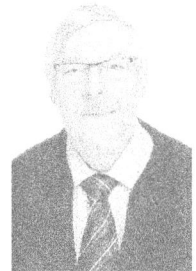

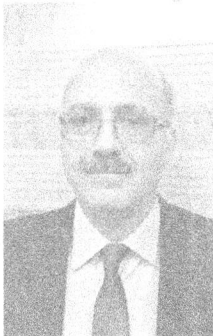

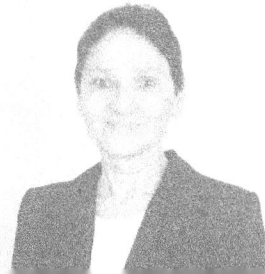

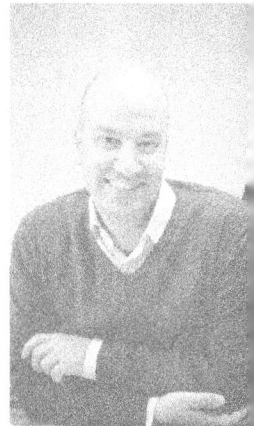

Cutaneous Melanoma
http://dx.doi.org/10.5772/intechopen.77684
Edited by Paweł Pietkiewicz

Contributors
Sunandana Chandra, Sarah E. Fenton, Jeffrey A. Sosman, Mariana Catalina De Anda Juárez, Ignatko Irina Vladimirovna, Strizhakov Alexander Nikolaevich, Wishrawana S. Sarathi Ratnayake, Mildred Acevedo-Duncan, Christopher A. Apostolatos, Pandurangan Ramaraj, Wei Gao, Bingjiang Lin, Valery Zakharov, Oleg O. Myakinin

Notice
Statements and opinions expressed in the chapters are these of the individual contributors and not necessarily those of the editors or publisher. No responsibility is accepted for the accuracy of information contained in the published chapters. The publisher assumes no responsibility for any damage or injury to persons or property arising out of the use of any materials, instructions, methods or ideas contained in the book.

First published in London, United Kingdom, 2020 by IntechOpen
IntechOpen is the global imprint of INTECHOPEN LIMITED, registered in England and Wales, registration number: 11086078, 7th floor, 10 Lower Thames Street, London, EC3R 6AF, United Kingdom
Printed in Croatia

British Library Cataloguing-in-Publication Data
A catalogue record for this book is available from the British Library

Additional hard and PDF copies can be obtained from orders@intechopen.com

Cutaneous Melanoma
Edited by Paweł Pietkiewicz
p. cm.
Print ISBN 978-1-78984-139-8
Online ISBN 978-1-78984-140-4
eBook (PDF) ISBN 978-1-78985-652-1

We are IntechOpen,
the world's leading publisher of
Open Access books
Built by scientists, for scientists

4,800+
Open access books available

123,000+
International authors and editors

135M+
Downloads

Our authors are among the

151
Countries delivered to

Top 1%
most cited scientists

12.2%
Contributors from top 500 universities

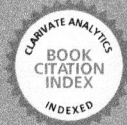

Interested in publishing with us?
Contact book.department@intechopen.com

Numbers displayed above are based on latest data collected.
For more information visit www.intechopen.com

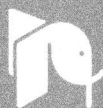

Meet the editor

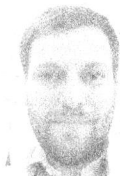

Dr Paweł Pietkiewicz is a board-certified dermatovenereologist (UEMS-EBDV). He earned his MD (2009) and summa cum laude PhD (2016) from Poznan University of Medical Sciences, Poznań, Poland, where he worked as a lecturer and a researcher. He is a recipient of Michael Hornstein Memorial EADV Scholarship (2015), SDF Grant (2015), Euroderm Excellence Grant (2015), SDS Grant (2017), BSPD Grant (2018), EADO Fellowship (2018) Sapienza University of Rome Fellowship (2018), and Eli Lilly Grant (2019). Dr Pietkiewicz was a winner of the Dermoscopy Excellence Challenge (2018) and AI Challenges (FotoFinder 2018, 2019; Canfield's DEXI - 2019). He has authored and co-authored over 100 manuscripts in dermatology and oncology. In 2018 he founded Polish Dermatoscopy Group for training medical specialists in skin cancer screening.

Contents

Preface

The American Cancer Society report states that skin cancer is the most common cancer of all cancer types with numbers exceeding all of the other cancers altogether. In spite of melanoma representing only about 1% of all skin cancers, this tumour is still responsible for most skin cancer deaths. The incidence of melanoma is steadily on the rise in respect to all thicknesses and stages. The peak incidence of the tumour is noted in late adulthood, yet according to US Surgeon General's 2018 report it is reported to be the third most common cancer in adolescents and young adults and the reason for this situation is multifactorial. A worrying trend is both outdoor and indoor tanning especially among young people and this is a main factor, even though the awareness of the need for sun protection is slightly on the rise due to social media campaigns. Recent reports indicate that the lifetime risk of developing a secondary melanoma has been underestimated for many years. This is a large-scale medical problem for the patients and a financial burden for the healthcare systems as many of these people will see the practitioners too late to avoid metastatic disease. Therefore, melanoma should be a matter of concern worldwide.

The book is divided into 3 sections. The first section focuses on the genetics and epigenetics of melanoma. Understanding the underlying mechanisms in tumour development and progression is pivotal for the development of new therapies. There has been massive progress in drug development for advanced stage disease in recent years. Presurgical biological treatment of a melanoma with dabrafenib/trametinib (BRAF/MEK inhibitors), nivolumab/ipilimumab and tissue agnostic anti-PD1 drug, pembrolizumab, showed promising outcomes in clinical trials regarding the recurrence rate in comparison to post-surgery treatment. Although IDO inhibitors are a disappointment, a whole new range of anti-cancer agents (eg. tavokinogene telsaplasmid, PKC inhibitors, and novel TLR9 agonists and anti-PD-1 drugs) give new hope to patients in with the advanced stage disease.

The second section of the book focuses on special melanoma scenarios. This section deals with the problem of melanoma in pregnancy. Many myths still surround this topic including the incidence, prognosis, available therapeutic options, possible complications, and prognosis. This sections also covers the subungual melanoma, as this clinical subtype tends to be a diagnostic challenge.

The third section follows the emerging trend of implementing mathematic models in skin cancer diagnosis. These models are being implemented nowadays in artificial intelligence deep-learning systems opening a new era of AI-assisted diagnostics. Although radiology was the first area affected by this process, I believe that the forthcoming years will bring it further to areas where visual imaging is crucial to establish the precise diagnosis - dermatology, ophthalmology, and pathology.

I hope that this book written by international experts will be a useful resource for both clinicians and researchers.

Paweł Pietkiewicz MD, PhD
FEACR, FEADO, FEADV, FEBDV, FESLD, FGILD, FIDS, FNYAS, FPDG, FPDS,
General and Oncological Surgery Clinic I,
Greater Poland Cancer Center,
Poznań, Poland

The Genetics and Epigenetics in Regulation of Melanoma Progression

Chapter 1

B-Raf-Mutated Melanoma

Sarah E. Fenton, Jeffrey A. Sosman and Sunandana Chandra

Abstract

Until fairly recently, treatment options for advanced melanoma have been relatively limited. Fortunately, the last decade has seen dramatic improvements in response rates and duration of overall survival after the introduction of checkpoint inhibitors and targeted therapies against mutations in the B-isoform of Raf (B-Raf) in metastatic or inoperable melanoma. This book chapter will discuss the role of wild type B-Raf in the cell, the changes induced by mutations in this protein, and current FDA approvals for targeted therapies against B-Raf, both as a monotherapy and in combination with MEK inhibitors. We will also summarize mechanisms of resistance against these targeted therapies as well as novel therapeutic regimens proposed to bypass resistance.

Keywords: melanoma, metastasis, B-Raf, MEK, targeted therapy, adjuvant

1. Introduction

Among all malignancies, melanoma is the fifth most common cancer in men and the sixth most common in women in the USA. With 91,270 new cases diagnosed in 2018 and 9320 fatalities, it has the fastest increase in incidence of any cancer worldwide [1–4]. Although the majority of cases are treated with excision, approximately 30% of patients will progress to metastatic disease [5]. On average, 60% of patients with local metastases will survive up to 5 years, while only 15% of patients with distant metastases will have similar survival rates [6]. Prior to 2011, the only approved treatment options for metastatic diseases were dacarbazine or high dose interleukin-2 (IL-2). These therapies were associated with response rates of 10–20% and rarely prolonged overall survival in the population of patients with metastatic melanoma [7–9]. Fortunately, the last decade has seen dramatic progress in melanoma treatment through the identification and targeting of mutations in the rapidly accelerated fibrosarcoma protein (Raf) that is an essential mediator of the mitogen-activated protein kinase (MAPK) pathway. First identified as an oncogene in 2002, Raf mutations have been found in melanoma, colorectal cancer, papillary thyroid carcinoma, non-small cell lung cancer, multiple myeloma, hairy cell leukemia, and specific subset of astrocytomas, to name a few malignancies [5]. Up to 50% of melanoma patients were found to carry a mutation in the B isoform of Raf (B-Raf), suggesting that targeted therapy was a promising strategy in the treatment of this disease [6, 10].

2. Role of B-Raf in the cell

Wild type B-Raf is a serine/threonine-specific protein kinase that acts as an important component of the MAPK pathway regulating cellular proliferation, survival, and differentiation. The B-Raf protein is composed of three main conserved regions that act by maintaining a closed conformation to autoinhibit protein function and to activate downstream pathway targets. Conserved region 1 (CR1) binds to conserved region 3 (CR3) to autoinhibit B-Raf function until activated by Ras. It also contains a zinc finger motif that aids in B-Raf docking at the cell membrane after activation. During activation, Ras binds to the CR1 domain allowing release of the bound CR3 domain. Conserved region 2 (CR2) acts to connect CR1 and CR3 and contains serine and tyrosine residues that are constitutively phosphorylated after Ras binding to help keep the protein in an open, active conformation and allow ATP binding. CR3 contains the enzymatic kinase domain of B-Raf, binding ATP and substrate proteins to catalyze the transfer of a phosphate group from ATP to the substrate, activating downstream signaling proteins. Importantly, this region also contains the valine amino acid at position 600, an amino acid that is often mutated resulting in the constitutive activation of B-Raf [11, 12].

B-Raf acts as a signaling protein in the Ras-Raf-Mek-Erk cascade, one of the most important oncogenic pathways in cancer. In wild type cells, extracellular growth factors and cytokines bind to transmembrane receptors on the cell's surface such as epidermal growth factor receptor (EGFR) and insulin like growth factor-1 receptor (IGF-1R). Intracellular phosphorylated sites on these receptors attract guanine nucleotide exchange factors (GEFs) such as SOS that bind to Ras and activate it by exchanging GDP for GTP. Once activated, Ras promotes the homo- and heterodimerization and activation of Raf kinases such as A-Raf, B-Raf and C-Raf. In turn, Raf kinases activate the MAP kinase pathway by phosphorylating MEK1 and MEK2. MEK proteins activate ERK 1 and 2 and the MAPK signaling pathway phosphorylates hundreds of downstream proteins [10, 13–16]. Importantly, activation of this pathway also sends inhibitory feedback towards upstream signaling components, which turn off signaling. This ultimately results in downregulation of Ras by ERK-dependent feedback [6]. Although the MAPK pathway is the most important downstream target of B-Raf, the JNK cascade, p38-MAPK pathway, and ERK-5 pathway have also been shown to be activated by B-Raf signaling [10].

3. Mutations in B-Raf that drive melanoma and their clinical significance

About 40–60% of melanomas will contain mutations in B-Raf at the V600 site, driving melanogenesis through upregulation of the Ras-Raf-Mek-ERK MAPK pathway [17]. Abnormal activation of the Ras-Raf-Mek Erk MAPK pathway is detected in approximately 90% of melanomas including the other genetic subsets such as Ras mutant, NF1 loss, and TWT [17]. Interestingly, other common mutations in melanoma, such as N-Ras, c-Kit, and NF1, also act through the MAPK pathway. B-Raf mutation alone is not considered sufficient to induce melanoma formation, as it has also been identified in benign and dysplastic nevi and can induce senescence [10, 18]. The vast majority (74–86%) of B-Raf mutations are substitutions of glutamic acid for valine at the 600th amino acid (V600E). However, substitutions of lysine for valine at amino acid 600 (V600K) in B-Raf is seen in 10–20% of melanomas and another 8% have other substations at the same site (V600M, V600D, and V600R) [6]. Case reports comparing the clinical significance of these different mutations show similar disease presentation and response to treatment [6, 9]. V600K mutations are more common in older patients and those with chronic sun exposure [9]. These B-Raf mutations occur in CR3 of the B-Raf protein and result in constitutive activation of the MAPK signaling pathway by destabilization of the inhibitory interaction between CR1 and CR3 through the introduction of a negatively charged or bulky amino acid at this site [10]. Mutations have also been identified in exon 15 (the region of DNA adjacent to V600), exon 11 and translocations involving the B-Raf gene in melanomas and melanoma cell lines. Despite the alternative locations of these mutations, some can also act to drive melanogenesis through activation of the MAPK pathway, but do not signal as a monomer like V600 mutant proteins and in some cases require Ras activation [9].

Clinically, B-Raf mutations are associated with patients that are younger at initial diagnosis (<50 years old), locations with largely intermittent sun exposure, earlier diagnosis of distant metastasis (56 versus 63 years old), increased incidence of brain metastasis, a higher number of nevi and lesions with a truncal location. B-Raf mutations are not induced by UV (sun) DNA damage. Most concerning, some studies suggest that these mutations have been associated with shortened median survival (5.7 versus 8.5 months). However, these studies are often not powered to examine survival [10, 19–21]. This may relate to their association with increased ulceration in the tumor, a prognostic factor that independently is associated with decreased survival [22]. Additionally, B-Raf mutations are more common in superficial spreading or nodular subtypes of melanoma [10].

4. Diagnosis and diagnostic testing

Clinical detection of B-Raf mutations is a powerful tool in the management of advanced melanoma, allowing clinicians to make decisions regarding treatment plans with targeted therapy versus alternatives such as immunotherapy. Molecular testing for B-Raf mutations is recommended by both the National Comprehensive Cancer Network (NCCN) and European Society for Medical Oncology (ESMO) guidelines in patients requiring systemic therapy [23–25]. This now includes most patients with stage III melanoma based on recent adjuvant trials. The sensitivity and specificity of the screening tests chosen is critical, as B-Raf detection and targeting is the only biomarker that can predict a therapeutic response to B-Raf inhibitor treatment in melanoma [23, 26]. Additionally, inappropriate treatment of B-Raf negative tumors with B-Raf inhibitors may be associated with tumor progression through paradoxical activation of the MAPK pathway based on numerous preclinical trials [27].

Due to advances in DNA sequencing, this method is being used more and more frequently as the initial method of mutation analysis. However, if there is not sufficient tissue or if rapid identification is needed diagnostic testing can be performed using immunohistochemistry with a VE1 monoclonal antibody to detect the V600E mutations. This method provides high sensitivity and is inexpensive. Unfortunately, it only detects this specific V600E mutation and misses other possible targets for B-Raf inhibitor therapy. Interpretation of immunohistochemistry by pathologists can also be subjective, making this method difficult to standardize. An alternative initial screening test is Sanger sequencing of the tumor DNA, often considered to be the gold standard. The tumor DNA is copied with amino acids attached to stop codons creating many copies of varying length that can be compared to determine the ultimate genetic sequence. This method is used less frequently, as a high ratio of mutant to wild type DNA is necessary to detect the B-Raf mutation and it has low sensitivity. If the immunohistochemistry or Sanger sequencing testing is negative it is often confirmed with pyrosequencing or RT-qPCR. Pyrosequencing is a method where DNA is sequenced using light tagged amino acids, allowing sequencing while the complementary DNA strand is being synthesized. This method is associated with a very high sensitivity for mutation detection; it also allows for quantification of mutated alleles in the tumor cell. However, pyrosequencing has a lower specificity than Sanger sequencing. Alternative confirmatory testing includes RT-qPCR, another highly sensitive method that is relatively rapid and inexpensive but relies on primer design and selection for mutation detection and may miss uncommon mutations. As Next Generation Sequencing (NGS) becomes less expensive and more readily available in the clinic, it is becoming a more common method of mutation detection, allowing high sensitivity and specificity as well as the detection of rare mutations [6, 28]. Finally, studies evaluating levels of circulating tumor DNA show promise in evaluating disease response and relapse [28].

The above testing modalities are all laboratory based and are used in diagnostic centers that have been certified by the Clinical Laboratory Improvement Amendments and have been reviewed by the US Centers for Medicare and Medicaid Services. However, there are two testing modalities that were developed in concert with the testing and approval of targeted therapies that are considered companion diagnostic tests. These have been reviewed by the FDA and approved for diagnostic testing prior to initiation of these specific drug therapies. B-Raf mutations are detected using two primary companion diagnostic tests, the cobas 4800 BRAF V600 Mutation Test (Roche Molecular Systems, Inc) and the THxID-BRAF kit (BioMerieux, Inc). Both RT-qPCR based, these tests were developed with vemurafenib plus cobimetinib and dabrafenib plus trametinib, respectively. Despite their high sensitivity, laboratory-based tests such as Sanger sequencing can be used to confirm negative results from companion diagnostic tests [28].

5. B-Raf inhibitor monotherapy

Given the frequency and importance of B-Raf in the development and progression of melanoma, interest in the development of B-Raf inhibitors was a high priority to all in the melanoma world. Three kinase inhibitors, vemurafenib, dabrafenib and encorafenib, are currently approved in the treatment of B-Raf V600-mutated melanoma. While they have been FDA approved in the treatment of B-Raf V600E and V600K-mutated melanomas, case studies and small trials suggest that these agents are also active in V600R mutants [6, 9]. However, based on published case reports, V600E mutations have improved response rates and longer progression-free survival after dabrafenib or vemurafenib treatment than other mutations [27].

Vemurafenib (PLX4032) is a B-Raf inhibitor that acts by binding to the ATP binding site in B-Raf, inhibiting the active form of the serine-threonine kinase [29, 30]. The BRIM3 trial was a phase III trial by Chapman et al. comparing vemurafenib targeted therapy (960 mg twice daily) with dacarbazine chemotherapy in 675 patients with untreated metastatic melanoma containing the B-Raf V600E or V600K mutation. The 6-month overall survival (OS) was 84% in the vemurafenib-treated group (95% confidence interval (CI) 78–89) versus 64% in the dacarbazine-treated group (95% CI, 56–73). Interim analysis showed a 63% reduction in the risk of death ($p < 0.001$) and a 74% reduction in the risk of either death or disease progression ($p < 0.001$) compared to dacarbazine. Overall response rates, a secondary endpoint, were 48% for vemurafenib and 5% for dacarbazine [31]. In follow up of this same population, McArthur et al. showed a median OS of 13.6 months in the vemurafenib-treated group (95% CI 12–15.2) versus 9.7 months in the dacarbazine-treated group (95% CI 7.9–12.8, $p < 0.001$). Progression-free survival (PFS) also improved with a median PFS of 6.9 months in the vemurafenib-treated group (95% CI 6.1–7) versus 1.6 months in the dacarbazine-treated group (95% CI 1.6–2.1, $p < 0.001$). Overall response rate increased with time to 57% in the vemurafenib group versus 9% in the dacarbazine group. Complete responses were seen in 6% of the vemurafenib-treated group versus 1% of the dacarbazine-treated group [32]. Based on these results, vemurafenib was the first approved drug for the treatment of B-Raf V600E and V600K-mutated advanced melanoma.

Dabrafenib (GSK2118436), another approved targeted therapy for the treatment of B-Raf V600-mutated melanoma, acts as a competitive inhibitor for ATP binding on the B-Raf protein and decreases its activity. Break-3 was a phase III trial by Hauschild et al. in which dabrafenib treatment (150 mg twice daily) was compared to dacarbazine administration. A total of 250 patients with previously untreated B-Raf V600E-mutated melanoma were enrolled. Dabrafenib therapy resulted in a median PFS of 5.1 months while the dacarbazine treatment group had a median PFS of 2.7 months. The hazard ratio for progression was 0.3 (95% CI 0.18–0.51, $p < 0.0001$). The OS hazard ratio was 0.61 (95% CI 0.25–1.48), suggesting significantly improved survival with dabrafenib treatment. About 50% of patients treated with dabrafenib had an objective response (95% CI 42.4–57.1) versus 7% with dacarbazine therapy (95% CI 1.8–15.5). Complete response was seen in 3% of patients treated with dabrafenib versus 2% of those treated with dacarbazine. Median time to response was 6.3 weeks (95% CI 6.1–6.3) with a median duration of response of 5.5 months. Patients that progressed on dacarbazine were allowed to cross over to treatment with dabrafenib, at the end of the study 44% of patients had crossed to dabrafenib treatment [33]. Based on these results, dabrafenib was approved by the FDA for treatment of B-Raf V600E-mutated advanced melanoma.

There has not been a direct head-to-head trial comparing dabrafenib and vemurafenib monotherapy in advanced melanoma with a B-Raf V600 mutation. However, extrapolating from the above trials suggests that they have very comparable clinical activity. Despite this, there is evidence suggesting that patients experience different drug-related toxicities. Vemurafenib was associated with toxicity requiring dose reduction due to grade 2 side effects in 38% of patients, while 28% of dabrafenib-treated patients required a dose reduction for grade 2 or greater side effects [32, 33]. Common toxicities of both drugs include rash, secondary skin malignancies (squamous cell carcinoma and keratoacanthomas), fatigue, arthralgia, and nausea. Vemurafenib was associated with higher rates of hepatic transaminitis, photosensitivity, and cutaneous hyperproliferative lesions; while, dabrafenib was associated with higher rates of pyrexia and chills. Despite the higher association with vemurafenib treatment, secondary skin hyperproliferative disorders and malignancies are seen with all B-Raf inhibitors. Median time to development of a squamous cell carcinoma after B-Raf inhibitor initiation is approximately 8 weeks and is seen in 20% of patients [10, 32]. These cutaneous side effects are primarily mediated by loss of feedback inhibition on the MAPK pathway after B-Raf suppression. In wild type cells, these B-Raf inhibitors accelerate B-Raf and C-Raf dimerization to activate the MAPK pathway. However, in B-Raf-mutated cells, signaling through negative feedback inhibition results in downregulation of MAPK signaling. After the addition of B-Raf inhibitors this negative feedback is lost, resulting in upregulation of MAPK signaling through C-Raf and Ras. Uncontrolled Ras activity has been associated with skin tumor formation, particularly squamous cell carcinomas. These patients are also at increased risk of new primary B-Raf wild type melanomas through similar mechanisms of action [6, 10].

B-Raf inhibition induces an overall response in approximately 50–60% of melanomas with B-Raf mutations. Predictors of response include B-Raf V600E mutations, higher PTEN levels at baseline (patients with deleted or mutant PTEN showed shorter PFS with dabrafenib therapy), initially increased levels of phosphorylated ERK followed by downregulation of phosphorylated ERK after treatment initiation, absence of MEK1p124 mutation, absence of CDKN2a gene deletion or chromosomal gains of the CCND1 gene [10]. Unfortunately, median progression-free survival with B-Raf targeted therapy is only 7 months [27, 31, 33]. Clinical factors that may be associated with a shorter PFS include an ECOG performance status of greater than 2, an elevated LDH at treatment initiation and M1C disease [10].

Even after clinical evidence of progression during treatment with vemurafenib or dabrafenib, studies suggest that continued treatment with B-Raf inhibitors may prolong survival through impedance of disease growth while preventing a disease flare that can be seen with cessation of treatment [10, 34, 35].

6. Combination therapy with B-Raf and MEK 1/2 inhibitors

Compared to the treatment modalities that were available prior to the development of targeted therapies, treatment with B-Raf inhibitors resulted in exceptional response rates and increases in overall survival. Investigation into inhibition at another downstream protein of the Ras-Raf-MEK-ERK MAPK pathway with MEK 1/2 inhibitors in the METRIC trials resulted in an overall response rate of approximately 30% and improved PFS of the oral selective MEK inhibitor trametinib when given orally (dose 2 mg) compared to treatment with dacarbazine in B-Raf-mutated melanoma [9, 36, 37]. Toxicities seen in the trial attributed to both drugs included rash, hypertension, diarrhea, edema, cardiac dysfunction, serum creatinine elevation, and ocular toxicities [10]. However, extrapolation from these studies and those of B-Raf inhibitors suggested that B-Raf inhibition was a more efficacious targeted therapy than MEK inhibition alone [38]. Relapse rates and side effect profiles with B-Raf inhibitor monotherapy were much higher than expected and were thought to be associated with reactivation of the MAPK pathway. For this reason, basic scientists and clinical investigators began combining B-Raf inhibitors with MEK inhibitors to block at two levels of this signaling pathway, intending to block any paradoxical activation after B-Raf inhibition [6]. Trametinib, cobimetinib, and bimimetinib are MEK inhibitors currently approved to be used in combination with B-Raf inhibitors in the treatment of advanced melanoma. Case reports also suggest that MEK inhibitors may be an effective therapy choice in patients with alternative mechanisms of MAPK activation, such as mutations in codons adjacent to that containing V600 [9].

The COMBI-DT, an initial phase II trial by Flaherty et al. evaluating dabrafenib and trametinib treatment in 247 patients with untreated B-Raf V600E- or V600K-mutated melanoma, found that dual targeted therapy (150 mg dabrafenib twice daily and 1 or 2 mg trametinib daily) resulted in a median PFS of 9.4 months versus 5.8 months for dabrafenib monotherapy. Median overall survival was 27.4 months for the combination therapy versus 20.2 months for the monotherapy. The hazard ratio for progression or death was 0.39 (95% CI 0.25–0.62, $p < 0.001$). Overall response was 76% in the dual therapy group compared to 54% with dabrafenib monotherapy ($p < 0.03$). Cutaneous side effects were significantly decreased with the addition of the MEK inhibitor [36, 37]. Following these results, phase III trials were performed showing similar outcomes. The COMBI-D phase III trial by Long et al. evaluated 423 patients with mutated B-Raf V600E or V600K advanced melanoma, who were treated with the combination of dabrafenib (150 mg twice daily) plus trametinib (2 mg daily) or dabrafenib alone. Median overall survival was 25.1 months in the combination group (95% CI 19.2–not reached) versus 18.7 months in the dabrafenib treatment group (95% CI 15.2–23.7, $p = 0.017$). Overall survival was 74% at 1 year and 51% at 2 years in the combination therapy group versus 68 and 42% in the monotherapy group. Median PFS was 11 months in the combination therapy group (95% CI 8–13.9) versus 8.8 months (95% CI 5.9–9.3, $p = 0.0004$). Rates of grade 3–4 adverse events were similar between both (32 versus 31%), pyrexia was the most common side effect with dabrafenib and trametinib combination therapy, while hyperkeratosis was the most common side effect in the dabrafenib alone group [39]. The COMBI-V study was a phase III trial by Robert et al. evaluating combination dabrafenib and trametinib therapy against vemurafenib monotherapy. A total of 704 patients with untreated mutant B-Raf V600E or V600K were randomized to receive dabrafenib (150 mg twice daily) with trametinib (2 mg once daily) versus vemurafenib (960 mg twice daily). Overall survival at 1 year was 72% in the combination therapy group (95% CI 67–77) versus 65% in the vemurafenib alone group (95% CI 59–70). Hazard ratio for death with combination therapy was 0.69 (95% CI 0.53–0.89, p = 0.005). Median PFS was 11.4 months in the combination therapy group and 7.3 months in the vemurafenib monotherapy group (HR 0.56, 95% CI 046–0.69, p = 0.001). Objective response rates were 64% in the combination therapy group and 51% in the monotherapy group (p < 0.001). Similar to the COMBI-D trial, rates of severe adverse events were comparable but rates of squamous cell carcinoma and other skin complications were significantly higher with vemurafenib monotherapy [40]. Based on these results, combination therapy with dabrafenib and trametinib was approved by the FDA for treatment of B-Raf-mutated V600E and -V600K advanced melanoma.

Another MEK inhibitor, cobimetinib, has also shown efficacy in combination with the B-Raf inhibitor vemurafenib in advanced melanoma. The coBRIM trial, a phase III trial by Larkin et al., studied 495 patients with untreated B-Raf-mutated V600E and -V600K advanced melanoma treated with vemurafenib (960 mg twice daily, continuously) and cobimetinib (60 mg daily for 21 days followed by 7 days off) versus vemurafenib alone. Median PFS was 9.9 months in the combination therapy group versus 6.2 months in the control group. The hazard ratio for death or progression was 0.51 (95% CI 0.39–0.68, p < 0.001). Overall response rates were 68% in the combination group versus 45% in the monotherapy treatment group (p < 0.001) with 10% of patients in the combination group achieving complete response (versus 4% in the vemurafenib alone group). Rates of adverse events trended toward higher occurrence in the combination therapy group; however, the difference was not significant (65% versus 59%) and rates of secondary skin cancers were lower in the combination therapy group [41]. A follow up study of the same patient population found a median PFS of 12.3 months (95% CI 9.5–13.4) in the combination therapy group versus 7.2 months in the vemurafenib group (95% CI 5.6-7.5, p < 0.0001). Median overall survival was 22.3 months for cobimetinib and vemurafenib treatment (95% CI 20.3–not estimable) versus 17.4 months for the vemurafenib group (95% CI 15-19.8, p = 0.005). Serious adverse events were seen in 37% of the combination treatment patients versus 28% of the monotherapy patients, the most significant of which were pyrexia and dehydration [42].

Second generation B-Raf inhibitors such as encorafenib were also tested in clinical trials in combination with MEK inhibitors. These drugs are associated with a 10× longer half-life than vemurafenib or dabrafenib [43]. Phase I/II trials have shown that combination therapy with encorafenib and the MEK inhibitor, binimetinib in B-Raf-mutated melanoma resulted in a median PFS of 11.3 months (95% CI 7.4–14.6) [44]. The COLUMBUS trial by Dummer et al. evaluated 577 patients with unresectable stage III or IV B-Raf V600E- or V600K-mutated mela-noma that were treatment naïve or had progressed on prior immunotherapy treated with encorafenib (450 mg daily) plus binimetinib (45 mg twice daily) or with encorafenib (300 mg daily) or vemurafenib (960 mg twice daily) monotherapy. Median PFS was 14.9 months (95% CI 11–18.5) in the combination encorafenib and binimetinib group versus 9.6 months in the encorafenib group (95% CI 7.5–14.8) and 7.3 months in the vemurafenib group (95% CI 5.6–8.2) (95% CI 0.41–0.71, HR 0.54, p < 0.0001). Overall responses were detected in 63% of patients in the combination therapy group versus 51% of patients with the encorafenib group and 40% of patients in the vemurafenib group [45]. Overall survival was 33.6 months (95% CI 24.4–39.2) in the combination therapy group versus 23.5 months (95%

CI 19.6–33.6) in the encorafenib group and 16.9 months in the vemurafenib group (95% CI 14–24.5) (HR 0.62, 95% CI 0.47–0.79, p < 0.0001) [46]. Adverse events in the combination therapy group included increased γ-glutamyltransferase, creatinine phosphokinase and hypertension. Encorafenib monotherapy was associated with palmoplantar erythrodysaesthesia syndrome, myalgia and arthralgia; while vemurafenib monotherapy was associated with arthralgia. Interestingly, combination therapy with encorafenib and binimetinib allowed a higher maximum tolerated dose of encorafenib, suggesting as with the other combinations of B-Raf and MEK inhibitors dual blockade of the MAPK pathway abrogates side effects associated with B-Raf inhibition alone. Fewer adverse events ultimately resulted in treatment discontinuation in the combination therapy group [45, 46]. Although it is difficult to compare end points between clinical trials, median PFS for encorafenib and binimetinib in the COLUMBUS trial was longer (14.9 months) than for either dabrafenib-trametinib in the COMBI-D (11 months) and COMBI-V (11.4 months) trials or for vemurafenib-cobimetinib in the coBRIM trial (12.3 months) [39, 40, 42, 45, 46]. This difference may be due to the longer half-life of encorafenib or it may also be the result of B-Raf treatment in a population of patients that did not all have access to immunotherapy due to local approved indications and regulations. This may have resulted in a group of patients on the COLUMBUS trial that was dissimilar to those studied in the other B-Raf inhibitor trials [45].

Overall, the above studies suggest that dual therapy with B-Raf and MEK inhibitors provides a longer PFS and increased overall response rates compared to B-Raf inhibition alone [38, 42, 47–50]. Most importantly, combination therapy is also associated with a modified side effect profile, particularly in those caused by reactivation of Ras and the MAPK pathway such as cutaneous squamous cell carcinomas [27]. Although the data suggest that encorafenib-binimetinib treatment may result in a slightly longer PFS, there is little direct evidence available to help clinicians pick between B-Raf/MEK inhibitor therapies [45, 46]. Therefore, the potential side effect profile may be helpful in guiding the decision. Approximately 50% of patients treated with dabrafenib and trametinib develop pyrexia, while 47% of patients treated with vemurafenib and cobimetinib develop significant photosensitivity [36, 40–42, 47]. Encorafenib and binimetinib dual therapy resulted in elevated γ-glutamyltransferase, creatinine phosphokinase, and hypertension [45, 46]. All combinations are associated with similar rates of MEK inhibitor-related toxicities such as serous retinopathy and left ventricular dysfunction [45, 46]. Other potential differences that may aid in picking therapy include the need to refrigerate trametinib and to take dabrafenib and trametinib on an empty stomach.

Monotherapy with a MEK inhibitor in B-Raf wild type tumors has been of great interest. Binimetinib treatment in melanomas with N-Ras mutations resulted in a PFS of 2.8 months (versus 1.5 months with dacarbazine), however overall survival was not improved [51, 52]. In vivo studies have also seen clinical activity from MEK inhibitor treatment in combination with CDK4/6 inhibitors, MDM2 antagonists, and PI3K/AKT inhibitors in melanoma [9]. Unfortunately, monotherapy with a MEK inhibitor such as trametinib after failure or B-Raf treatment showed no response [6, 10].

7. Adjuvant therapy with B-Raf inhibition

The above studies evaluated combined targeted therapy in advanced melanoma, where the patients were either not surgical candidates or had metastatic disease. However, investigators have also evaluated whether adjuvant targeted therapy after surgical resection may result in increased progression-free or overall survival.

The COMBI-AD trial by Long et al. was a phase III trial, where 870 patients with resected stage IIIA, IIB and IIIC B-Raf V600E- or V600K-mutated melanoma were randomly assigned to placebo or treatment with dabrafenib (150 mg twice daily) and trametinib (2 mg daily). Estimated relapse free survival rates at 3 years were 58% in the treatment group versus 39% in the placebo group (HR for death 0.47, 95% CI 0.39–0.58, p < 0.001). Overall survival at 3 years was 86% in the treatment group versus 77% in the placebo group (HR for death 0.57, 95% CI 0.42–0.79, p = 0.0006). Combination treatment with dabrafenib and trametinib also resulted in increased metastasis-free survival and lower rates of relapse. Despite the 53% improvement in relapse free survival and 43% improvement in overall survival, these improvements must be weighed against the 26% discontinuation rate due to adverse events (most frequently pyrexia and fatigue) [53]. Hauschild et al. confirmed these results in an extended follow up, evaluating relapse free survival rates at 3 and 4 years for dabrafenib and trametinib co-therapy versus placebo. At 3 years, relapse free survival rates were 59% for combination therapy (95% CI 55–64%) versus 40% in the placebo arm (95% CI 35–45%). At 4 years, relapse free survival rates were 54% for combination therapy (95% CI 49–59%) versus 38% in the placebo arm (95% CI 34–44%) [54]. Single agent vemurafenib (960 mg twice daily) as adjuvant therapy was also studied after resection in patients with stage IIC, IIIA, IIIB, or IIIC melanoma. Treatment resulted in a substantial but not significant increase in disease-free survival [55]. These new data suggest that B-Raf and MEK inhibition not only play an important role in the treatment of metastatic melanoma, but they also may provide benefit to patients with stage III disease after surgical resection.

8. B-Raf targeted therapy in brain metastases

As discussed previously, B-Raf inhibitor therapy is an effective treatment option for patients with inoperable or metastatic melanoma. Unfortunately, melanoma has one of the highest cerebral tropisms of any malignancy. Approximately 20% of stage IV patients have brain metastases at time of diagnosis and up to 40–50% of patients with stage IV melanoma will ultimately develop intracranial disease [56]. This development contributes significantly to mortality in 20–54% of metastatic melanoma patients; and once brain metastases are diagnosed, median survival decreases to 4–5 months [56–58]. Therefore, in evaluating the efficacy of targeted and immunotherapies in advanced melanoma, it is important to evaluate whether these agents are active in the central nervous system. The BREAK-MB trial showed that dabrafenib (150 mg twice a day) had an acceptable safety profile and induced a response in the metastatic brain lesions of 39% of B-Raf V600E mutant advanced melanoma if no prior local therapy had been used and in 31% of patients with prior local therapy. Median progression-free survival was 16 weeks and median overall survival was 31 weeks [59]. The COMBI-MB trial by Davies et al. was a phase II trial of dabrafenib (150 mg twice a day) and trametinib (2 mg daily) in 125 patients with V600 mutant melanoma. About 58% of patients with asymptomatic brain metastases and no prior therapy showed a response (95% CI 46–69) with a median progression-free survival of 5.6 months (95% CI 5.3–7.4) and a median overall survival of 10.8 months (95% CI 9.7–19.6). About 56% of patients who had received prior therapy showed a response with a median PFS of 7.2 month (95% CI 1.7–6.5), while 59% of patients with symptomatic brain metastases showed a response with a median PFS of 5.5 months (95% CI 2.8–7.3). About 44% of patients with V600D/K/R mutations responded to dabrafenib and trametinib with a median PFS of 4.2 months (95% CI 1.7–6.5) [60]. Vemurafenib has been studied in a phase 2 trial with similar results [57, 58]. Interestingly, these trials show that there is a decreased response in the brain lesions when compared to extracranial lesions after B-Raf inhibition and overall the duration of response is approximately 50% that of extracranial sites, which may be due to higher concentrations of drug at the extracranial tumor site [61, 62].

Unfortunately, investigators have also found that the brain is a frequent site of disease recurrence or metastases after B-Raf inhibition [58]. This is thought to be related to signaling changes in the metastatic cell. MAPK downregulation is associated with upregulation of the PI3K/AKT pathway. Increased signaling through this pathway is often found in brain metastases [62, 63]. Therefore, it is also important to continue to investigate optimal treatment for intracranial disease after treatment with B-Raf inhibitors.

9. Mechanisms of resistance

Initial response rates to B-Raf inhibitors in B-Raf-mutated melanoma ranged between 50 and 70%, suggesting that 30–50% of these tumors have a mechanism of primary resistance prior to therapy. Additionally, approximately 50% of patients treated with B-Raf targeted therapy develop resistance within 1 year and only 10% of patients will respond to combination B-Raf and MEK targeted therapy for at least 3 years [10]. On average, resistance to B-Raf inhibition occurs after 6–8 months of treatment, although this is prolonged with dual MEK inhibition [38]. Evaluation of tumor samples after the development of B-Raf inhibitor resistance showed 38% of the mechanisms of resistance were non-genomic in origin, while 56% were due to both genomic and non-genomic changes [64]. About 79% of these mechanisms are associated with MAPK signaling reactivation [38]. Adjusting treatment regimens to address B-Raf inhibitor resistance is made even more difficult by the finding that several resistance mechanisms often coexist within the same tumor or between different tumor sites in patients treated with B-Raf inhibitors [27, 38].

Although mechanisms of primary resistance have been defined, it is difficult to conclusively establish that there was no response to treatment. Almost all patients with B-Raf-mutated melanoma respond initially to B-Raf inhibition; however, the duration of response is so short that there is evidence of progression at the time of disease evaluation. Alterations in the MAPK pathway such as predominance of signaling through C-Raf or the PI3K pathway increases immunity to B-Raf inhibition. NF1 is a tumor suppression that acts to inhibit Ras, and loss of NF1 function leads to constitutive Ras activation and activation of the MAPK pathway irrelevant of B-Raf inhibition. Through similar signaling changes, alterations in the PI3k-AKT-mTOR pathway (such as loss of function in PTEN) lead to constitutive activation of AKT and cell survival. Alterations in the RB1 pathway through mutations in cyclin D1, CDK4, or CDK6 can also lead to cell cycle progression irrelevant of B-Raf signaling [6].

Mechanisms of secondary resistance that develop after treatment with B-Raf inhibitors predominantly occur through changes allowing MAPK signaling despite B-Raf inhibition. Signaling through the MAPK pathway can be restored through N-Ras or MEK1/2 activating mutations. Upregulation and activation of the receptor tyrosine kinases and the PI3K-AKT-mTOR pathway (through IGF1-R, PDGFRβ, MET, mTORC1/2, EGFR, and ERBB3) can also activate MAPK signaling regardless of B-Raf inhibition. These changes have been identified in cell lines and in biopsies from the tumors of B-Raf inhibitor-treated patients after progression. Feedback activation of EGFR following B-Raf inhibition causes resistance through deactivation of MIG6 and increased expression of SOX10, restoring downstream signaling. But the most important pathways effect the B-Raf V600 molecule themselves, including alternative splicing of the B-Raf V600E protein resulting in loss of the RAS binding domain and decreased sensitivity to the inhibitor as well as amplification of the B-RAF V600 gene inducing an overabundance of ligand. Copy number amplification of the B-Raf mutation can result in drug saturation and lead to dimerization despite inhibitor exposure, allowing downstream activation. Upregulation of C-Raf can increase signaling through a similar mechanism. MAP3K8 encodes COT, a protein that phosphorylates MEK independently of Raf signaling. Mutations in MAP3K8 have been identified in resistant tumors. Shifts in cellular metabolism to favor oxidative metabolism through increased expression of PGC1alpha have also been associated with B-Raf inhibition [6, 10]. Increased signaling through the YAP pathway and escape from cell death through upregulation of Bcl-XL have been identified in resistant cells after treatment with B-Raf inhibitors [9]. Mutations in the PI3K-AKT pathway (either through positive regulation of the pathway or negative regulation of its inhibitors PIK3R2 or PHLPP1) can upregulate signaling through this pathway, allowing cell survival despite B-Raf inhibition [6, 10]. The tumor microenvironment can also upregulate MAPK signaling through increased MAPK signaling in melanoma-associated fibroblasts after B-Raf inhibitor exposure. These fibroblasts act to promote matrix formation and remodeling, creating a protective environment for the tumor cell [38, 65]. In a study of 132 melanoma samples collected after the development of B-Raf inhibitor resistance, 20% had a N-Ras/K-Ras mutation, 16% had developed a B-Raf splice variant, 13% showed B-Raf amplification, 7% had a MEK1/2 mutation, and 11% developed an alteration in a non-MAPK signaling pathway [66]. Combined treatment with B-Raf and MEK inhibitors has shown development of resistance through similar mechanisms [67]. In fact, resistance after treatment with combination therapy is more often mediated through MAPK signaling reactivation than after treatment with B-Raf inhibitor monotherapy (82 versus 50%) [66, 67].

Due to the relative high rate of primary and secondary resistance to B-Raf inhibitors, alternative dosing schedules are being studied to see if these slow the rate of treatment escape. Intermittent dosing schedules show some promise in increasing the average time to progression for B-Raf-mutated melanomas treated with B-Raf inhibition [10].

10. Future directions

In vivo data and studies involving patient tumor samples have found that soon after B-Raf inhibitor initiation, immune activation is enhanced in the tumor microenvironment through multiple mechanisms [6]. The microphthalmia-associated transcription factor (MITF) is activated by MAPK signaling to suppress the expression of melanocyte-lineage antigens. Blockade of this pathway with B-Raf inhibitors upregulates expression of these melanoma-specific antigens, increasing the immune system's ability to recognize and target tumor cells. By the time tumor progression is noted on B-Raf inhibitors, these markers are usually downregulated and suppressed. B-Raf inhibition is also associated with an increase in tumor infiltrating lymphocytes early after treatment initiation. Finally, B-Raf inhibition often results in decreases in the immunosuppressive cytokines interleukin (IL)-6 and IL-8. Associated with a better tumor response to B-Raf inhibition, these findings suggest that adding immunotherapy or employing immunotherapy somewhere in the treatment course may be beneficial [38, 68]. Mouse studies have also demonstrated that treatment with dabrafenib, trametinib, and an anti-PD1 immunotherapy resulted in improved outcomes compared to either therapy alone [38, 69]. Attempts at combining vemurafenib and ipilimumab have been terminated due to poor tolerability including fulminant hepatitis [6]. However, clinical investigators have been evaluating responses to alternative combinations of B-Raf and MEK inhibitors with checkpoint inhibitors. Ribas et al. performed a phase I study combining dabrafenib, trametinib, and an anti-PD-L1 monoclonal antibody MEDI4736. Six patients with B-Raf-mutated advanced melanoma were treated with either MED14736 (3 or 10 mg/kg IV every 2 weeks), dabrafenib (150 mg twice daily) and trametinib (2 mg daily), or trametinib alone. Thrombocytopenia was the main dose limiting toxicity identified. About 100% of patients had a response to combination therapy [70]. Another phase I trial combining atezolizumab, an anti-PD-L1 antibody (800 mg every 2 weeks), cobimetinib (60 mg daily) and vemurafenib (960 mg twice a day for the first 21 days, then 720 mg daily) in 34 patients with B-Raf-mutated advanced melanoma found that this combination resulted in a manageable and reversible safety profile. Partial or complete responses were detected in 85.3% of patients [71, 72]. Combination therapy in a phase 1/2 trial with pembrolizumab (2 mg/kg every 3 weeks), dabrafenib (150 mg twice daily) and trametinib (2 mg daily) in 15 patients with advanced B-Raf mutant melanoma found manageable and reversible dose limiting toxicities and adverse events. About 60% of patients had a complete or partial response [73]. Finally, a phase I trial of pembrolizumab (2 mg/kg every 3 weeks), dabrafenib (150 mg twice a day), and trametinib (2 mg daily) was compared with dabrafenib/trametinib treatment in 60 patients with B-Raf-mutated metastatic melanoma found a median PFS in the triple therapy group of 16 months (95% CI 8.6–21.5) versus 10.3 months in the dual therapy group (95% CI 7–15.6, HR 0.66, p-0.04287). Rates of response were also more durable, 60% of patients on triple therapy had responses that lasted over 18 months compared to 26% dual therapy [74]. Many other clinical trials are ongoing evaluating the clinical benefit of treatment with combinations of B-Raf inhibitors and immunotherapy (NCT02130466, NCT02967692, NCT02908672, NCT02858921, NCT02224781, NCT01656642, NCT01673854, NCT01940809, NCT02631447, NCT03235245, and NCT02902042). Some tissue and mouse studies indicate that MEK inhibition impairs T cell proliferation and localization to the tumor tissue, suggesting combination therapies with MEK inhibitors and immunotherapy may not be synergistic. However, these findings have not been recapitulated in clinical trials (NCT01767454) [9].

Additionally, immunotherapy monotherapy trials have shown that treatment with nivolumab and pembrolizumab in B-Raf mutant and B-Raf inhibitor refractory disease is associated with promising results [9, 38]. A small study of 19 pts showed an improved overall survival with a transition of therapy from vemurafenib to ipilimumab within 4 months of starting [10].

In addition to combination therapies, clinicians and scientists have been evaluating alternative methods to avoid or overcome resistance mechanisms after B-Raf therapy. These include using Bcl inhibitors to prevent cell escape through the YAP pathway, autophagy inhibitors that act through Bcl-2m Bcl-XL and Bcl-w, mTor inhibitors, ERK inhibitors, additional MAPK inhibitors, or Jak inhibitors to bypass other mechanisms of survival [9, 10].

11. Conclusions

Compared to other currently approved therapies for advanced melanoma, B-Raf inhibitors are associated with a rapid onset of tumor regression, often within 1–2 weeks of treatment [9]. The speed of response is particularly beneficial in patients with a rapidly progressive or high burden of disease, as well as those with a poor performance status. The ECOG 6134 trial (NCT02224781) is accruing in an attempt to answer whether initial treatment with checkpoint inhibitors or targeted therapy is more beneficial. This is a crucial study for which an answer will provide vital evidence for the sequencing of immunotherapy and B-Raf targeted therapy.

The introduction of B-Raf inhibitors has been an important component in the revolution of melanoma treatment that has occurred in the last decade. Vemurafenib, dabrafenib, and encorafenib in combination with MEK inhibitors such as cobimetinib, trametinib, and binimetinib, have resulted in unprecedented overall responses and increases in survival. Combination therapy has also improved patient outcomes and decreased the likelihood of significant side effects such as new cutaneous malignancies. Testing for B-Raf mutations and treatment with B-Raf inhibitors is now standard of care in oncology clinics throughout the world. However, there is still significant ongoing work in management of tumor resistance mechanisms and combination and/or sequential regimens are being studied with immuno-oncologic agents, as an example, to try to further boost the efficacy, while maintaining an acceptable safety and tolerability profile.

Author details

Sarah E. Fenton, Jeffrey A. Sosman and Sunandana Chandra*
Division of Hematology and Oncology, Northwestern University, Chicago, IL, USA

*Address all correspondence to: sunandana.chandra@northwestern.edu

IntechOpen

References

[1] Mansfield AS, Nevala WK, Lieser EA, Leontovich AA, Markovic SN. The immunomodulatory effects of bevacizumab on systemic immunity in patients with metastatic melanoma. Oncoimmunology. 2013;**2**(5):e24436

[2] Emmett MS, Dewing D, Pritchard-Jones RO. Angiogenesis and melanoma—From basic science to clinical trials. American Journal of Cancer Research. 2011;**1**(7):852-868

[3] Siegel RL, Miller KD, Jemal A. Cancer statistics. CA: A Cancer Journal for Clinicians. 2016;**66**(1):7-30

[4] Siegel RL, Miller KD, Jemal A. Cancer statistics. CA: A Cancer Journal for Clinicians. 2018;**68**(1):7-30

[5] Tas F. Metastatic behavior in melanoma: Timing, pattern, survival, and influencing factors. Journal of Oncology. 2012;**2012**:647684

[6] Spagnolo F, Ghiorzo P, Orgiano L, Pastorino L, Picasso V, Tornari E, et al. BRAF-mutant melanoma: Treatment approaches, resistance mechanisms and diagnostic strategies. OncoTargets and Therapy. 2015;**8**:157-168

[7] Carbone PP, Costello W. Eastern cooperative oncology group studies with DTIC (NSC-45388). Cancer Treatment Reports. 1976;**60**(2):193-198

[8] Atkins MB, Lotze MT, Dutcher JP, Fisher RI, Weiss G, Margolin K, et al. High-dose recombinant interleukin 2 therapy for patients with metastatic melanoma: Analysis of 270 patients treated between 1985 and 1993. Journal of Clinical Oncology. 1999;**17**(7):2105-2116

[9] Luke JJ, Flaherty KT, Ribas A, Long GV. Targeted agents and immunotherapies: Optimizing outcomes in melanoma. Nature Reviews. Clinical Oncology. 2017;**14**(8):463-482

[10] Carlino MS, Long GV, Kefford RF, Rizos H. Targeting oncogenic BRAF and aberrant MAPK activation in the treatment of cutaneous melanoma. Critical Reviews in Oncology/Hematology. 2015;**96**(3):385-398

[11] Morrison DK, Cutler RE. The complexity of Raf-1 regulation. Current Opinion in Cell Biology. 1997;**9**(2):174-179

[12] Roskoski R Jr. RAF protein-serine/threonine kinases: Structure and regulation. Biochemical and Biophysical Research Communications. 2010;**399**(3):313-317

[13] Roskoski R Jr. Targeting oncogenic Raf protein-serine/threonine kianses in human cancers. Pharmacological Research. 2018;**135**:239-258

[14] Simanshu DK, Nissley DV, McCormick F. RAS proteins and their regulators in human disease. Cell. 2017;**170**(1):17-33

[15] Holderfield M, Deuker MM, McCormick F, McMahon M. Targeting RAF kinases for cancer therapy: BRAF-mutated melanoma and beyond. Nature Reviews. Cancer. 2014;**14**(7):455-467

[16] Roskoski R Jr. ERK1/2 MAP kinases: Structure, function, and regulation. Pharmacological Research. 2012;**66**(2):105-143

[17] Davies H, Bignell GR, Cox C, Stephens P, Edkins S, Clegg S, et al. Mutations of the BRAF gene in human cancer. Nature. 2002;**417**(6892):949-954

[18] Pollock PM, Harper UL, Hansen KS, Yudt LM, Stark M, Robbins CM, et al. High frequency of BRAF mutations in nevi. Nature Genetics. 2003;**33**(1):19-20

[19] Long GV, Menzies AM, Nagrial AM, Haydu LE, Hamilton AL, Mann GJ, et al. Prognostic and clinicopathologic associations of oncogenic BRAF in metastatic melanoma. Journal of Clinical Oncology. 2011;**29**(10):1239-1246

[20] Ribas A, Flaherty KT. BRAF targeted therapy changes the treatment paradigm in melanoma. Nature Reviews. Clinical Oncology. 2011;**24**:426-433

[21] Hugdahl E, Kalvenes MB, Puntervoll HE, Ladstein RG, Akslen LA. BRAF-V600E expression in primary nodular melanoma is associated with aggressive tumour features and reduced survival. British Journal of Cancer. 2016;**114**(7):801-808

[22] Ellerhorst JA, Greene VR, Ekmekcioglu S, Sarneke CL, Johnson MM, Cooke CP, et al. Clinical correlates of NRAS and BRAF mutations in primary human melanoma. Clinical Cancer Research. 2011;**17**(2):229-235

[23] National Comprehensive Cancer Network (NCCN). Practice Guidelines in Oncology: Melanoma Version 1. Available from: https://www.nccn.org/professionals/physician_gls/pdf/melanoma.pdf [Accessed: 2017]

[24] Dummer R, Hauschild A, Lindenblatt N, Pentheroudakis G, Keilholz U. Cutaneous melanoma: ESMO clinical practice guidelines for diagnosis, treatment, and follow-up. Annals of Oncology. 2016;(Suppl 5): 126-132

[25] Garbe C, Peris K, Hauschild A, Saiag P, Middleton J, Bastholt L, et al. Diagnosis and treatment of melanoma. European consensus-based interdisciplinary guideline-update 2016. European Journal of Cancer. 2016;**63**:201-217

[26] Dummer R, Hauschild A, Lindenblatt N, Pentheroudakis G,

Keilholz U. Cutaneous melanoma: ESMO clinical practice guidelines for diagnosis, treatment and follow-up. Annals of Oncology. 2017;**26**:v126-v132

[27] Menzies AM, Long GV. Systemic treatment for BRAF-mutant melanoma: Where do we go next? The Lancet Oncology. 2014;**15**(9):e371-e381

[28] Cheng L, Lopez-Beltran A, Massari F, MacLennan GT, Montironi R. Molecular testing for BRAF mtuations to inform melanoma treatment decisions: A move toward precision medicine. Modern Pathology. 2018;**31**(1):24-38

[29] Tsai J, Lee JT, Wang W, Zhang J, Cho H, Mamo S, et al. Discovery of a selective inhibitor of oncogenic B-Raf kinase with potent antimelanoma activity. Proceedings of the National Academy of Sciences. 2008;**105**(8):3041-3046

[30] Bollag G, Hirth P, Tsai J, Zhang J, Ibrahim PN, Cho H, et al. Clinical efficacy of a RAF inhibitor needs broad target blockade in BRAF-mutant melanoma. Nature. 2010;**467**(7315):596-599

[31] Chapman PB, Hauschild A, Robert C, Haanen JB, Ascierto P, Larkin J, et al. Improved survival with vemurafenib in melanoma with BRAF V600E mutation. The New England Journal of Medicine. 2011;**364**(26):2507-2516

[32] McArthur GA, Chapman PB, Robert C, Larkin J, Haanen JB, Dummer R, et al. Safety and efficacy of vemurafenib in BRAFV600E and BRAFV600K mutation-positive melanoma (BRIM-3): Extended follow-up of a phase 3, randomised, open-label study. The Lancet Oncology. 2014;**15**(3):323-332

[33] Hauschild A, Grob JJ, Demidov LV, JOuary T, Gutzmer R, Millward M, et al. Dabrafenib in BRAF-mutated

metastatic melanoma: A multicentre, open-label, phase 3 randomised controlled trial. Lancet. 2012;**380**(9839):358-365

[34] Chan MM, Haydu LE, Menzies AM, Azer MW, Klein O, Lyle M, et al. The nature and management of metastatic melanoma after progression on BRAF inhibitors: Effects of extended BRAF inhibition. Cancer. 2014;**120**(20):3142-3153

[35] Carlino MS, Gowrishankar K, Saunders CA, Pupo GM, Snoyman S, Zhang XD, et al. Antiproliferative effects of continued mitogen-activated protein kinase pathway inhibition following acquired resistance to BRAF and/ or MEK inhibition in melanoma. Molecular Cancer Therapeutics. 2013;**12**(7):1332-1342

[36] Flaherty KT, Robert C, Hersey P, Nathan P, Garbe C, Milhelm M, et al. Improved survival with MEK inhibition in BRAF-mutated melanoma. The New England Journal of Medicine. 2012;**367**(2):107-114

[37] Flaherty KT, Infante JR, Daud A, Gonzalez R, Kefford RF, Sosman J, et al. Combined BRAF and MEK inhibition in melanoma with BRAF V600 mutations. The New England Journal of Medicine. 2012;**367**(18):1694-1703

[38] Welsh SJ, Rizos H, Scolyer RA, Long GV. Resistance to combination BRAF and MEK inhibition in metastatic melanoma: Where to next? European Journal of Cancer. 2016;**62**:76-85

[39] Long GV, Stroyakovskiy D, Gogas H, Levchenko E, de Graud F, Larkin J, et al. Dabrafenib and trametinib versus dabrafenib and placebo for Val600 BRAF-mutant melanoma: A multicentre, double-blind, phase 3 randomised controlled trial. Lancet. 2015;**386**(9992):444-451

[40] Robert C, Karaszewska B, Schachter J, Rutkowski P, Mackiewicz A, Stroiakovski D, et al. Imrproved overall survival in melanoma with combined dabrafenib and trametinib. The New England Journal of Medicine. 2015;**372**(1):30-39

[41] Larkin J, Ascierto PA, Dreno B, Atkinson V, Liszkay G, Maio M, et al. Combined vemurafenib and cobimetinib in BRAF-mutated melanoma. The New England Journal of Medicine. 2014;**371**(20):1867-1876

[42] Ascierto PA, McArthur GA, Dreno B, Atkinson V, Liszkay G, Di Giacomo AM, et al. Cobimetinib combined with vemurafenib in advanced BRAF(V600)-mutant melanoma (coBRIM): Updated efficacy results from a randomized, double-blind, phase 3 trial. The Lancet Oncology. 2016;**17**(9):1248-1260

[43] Delord JP, Robert C, Nyakas M, McArthur GA, Kudchakar R, Mahipal A, et al. Phase I dose-escalation and -expansion study of the BRAF inhibitor encorafenib (LGX818) in metastatic BRAF-mutant melanoma. Clinical Cancer Research. 2017;**23**(18):5339-5384

[44] Sullivan RJ, Weber JS, Patel SP, Dummer R, Miller WH, Cosgrive D, et al. A phase Ib/II study of BRAF inhibitor (BRAFi) encorafenib (ENCO) plus MEK inhibitor (MEKi) binimetinib (BINI) in cutaneous melanoma patients naïve to BRAFI treatment. ASCO Meeting. 2015;**33**:9007

[45] Dummer R, Ascierto PA, Gogas HJ, Arance A, Mandala M, Liszkay G, et al. Encorafenib plus binimetinib versus vemurafenib or encorafenib in patients with BRAF-mutant melanoma (COLUMBUS): A multicentre, open-label, randomized phase 3 trial. The Lancet Oncology. 2018;**19**(5):603-615

[46] Dummer R, Ascierto PA, Gogas HJ, Arance A, Mandala M, Liszkay G, et al. Overall survival in patients with BRAF-mutant melanoma receiving encorafenib plus binimetinib versus vemurafenib or encorafenib (COLUMBUS): A multicentre, open-label, randomized, phase 3 trial. The Lancet Oncology. 2018;**19**(10):1315-1327

[47] Long GV, Stroyakovskiy D, Gogas H, Levchenko E, de Braud F, Larkin J, et al. Combined BRAF and MEK inhibition versus BRAF inhibition alone in melanoma. The New England Journal of Medicine. 2014;**371**(20):1877-1888

[48] Long GV, Flaherty KT, Stroyakovskiy D, Gogas H, Levchenko E, de Braud F, et al. Dabrafenib plus trametinib versus dabrafenib monotherapy in patients with metastatic BRAF V600E/K-mutant melanoma: Long-term survival and safety analysis of a phase 3 study. Annals of Oncology. 2017;**28**:1631-1639

[49] Robert C, Karaszewska B, Schachter J, Rutkowski P, Mackiewicz A, Stroyakovskiy D, et al. Three-year estimate of overall survival in COMBI-v, a randomized phase 3 study evaluating first-line dabrafenib (D)+trametinib (T) in patients (pts) with unresectable or metastatic BRAF V600E/K–mutant cutaneous melanoma. Annals of Oncology. 2016;**27**:LBA40

[50] Long GV, Weber JS, Infante JR, Kim KB, Daud A, Gonzalez R, et al. Overall survival and durable responses in patients with BRAF V600-mutant metastatic melanoma receiving dabrafenib combined with trametinib. Journal of Clinical Oncology. 2016;**34**:871-878

[51] Ascierto PA, Schadendorf D, Berking C, Agarwala SS, van Herpen CM, Queirolo P, et al. MEK162 for patients with advanced melanoma horbouring NRAS or Val600 BRAF mutations: A non-randomised, open-label phase 2 study. The Lancet Oncology. 2013;**14**(3):249-256

[52] Dummer R, Shadendorf D, Ascierto PA, Fernandez AMA, Dutriaux C, Maio M, et al. Results of NEMO: A phase III trial of binimetinib (BINI) versus dacarbazine (DTIC) in NRAS-mutant cutaneous melanoma. Journal of Clinical Oncology. 2016;**34**(Suppl):9500

[53] Long GV, Hauschild A, Santinami M, Atkinson V, Mandala M, Chiarion-Sileni V, et al. Adjuvant dabrafenib plus trametinib in stage III BRAF-mutated melanoma. The New England Journal of Medicine. 2017;**377**(19):1813-1823

[54] Hauschild A, Dummer R, Schadendorf D, Santinami M, Atkinson V, Mandala M, et al. Longer follow-up confirms relapse-free survival benefit with adjuvant dabrafenib plus trametinib in patients with resected BRAF V600-mutant stage III melanoma. Journal of Clinical Oncology. 2018;**22**:JCO1801219

[55] Lewis K, Maio M, Demidov L, Mandala M, Ascierto PA, Herbert C, et al. A randomized, double-blind, placebo-controlled study of adjuvant vemura1fenib in patients with completely resected BRAF V600+ melanoma at high risk for recurrence. ESMO 2017 Congress. Abstract LBA7_PR. Presented September 11, 2017

[56] Davies MA, Liu P, McIntyre S, Kim KB, Papadopoulos N, Hwu WJ, et al. Prognostic factors for survival in melanoma patients with brain metastases. Cancer. 2011;**117**(8):1687-1696

[57] McArthur GA, Maio M, Arance A, Nathan P, Blank C, Avril MF, et al. Vemurafenib in metastatic melanoma patients with brain metastases: An open-label, single-arm, phase 2, multicentre study. Annals of Oncology. 2017;**28**(3):634-641

[58] Foppen G, Boogerd W, Blank CU, van Thienen JV, Haanen JB, Brandsma D. Clinical and radiological response of BRAF inhibition and MEK inhibition in patients with brain metastases from BRAF-mutated melanoma. Melanoma Research. 2018;**28**(2):126-133

[59] Long GV, Trefzer U, Davies MA, Kefford F, Ascierto PA, Chapman PB, et al. Dabrafenib in patients with Val600Glu or Val600Lys *BRAF*-mutant melanoma metastatic to the brain (BREAK-MB): A multicentre, open-label, phase 2 trial. The Lancet Oncology. 2012;**13**(11):1087-1095

[60] Davies MA, Saiag P, Robert C, Grob JJ, Flaherty KT, Arance A, et al. Dabrafenib plus trametinib in patients with *BRAF*^V600^-mutant melanoma brain metastases (COMBI-MB): A multicentre, multicohort, open-label, phase 2 trial. The Lancet Oncology. 2017;**18**(7):863-873

[61] Tawbi HA, Boutros C, Kok D, Robert C, McArthur G. New era in the management of melanoma brain metastases. American Society of Clinical Oncology Educational Book. 2018;**38**:741-750

[62] Davies MA, Stemke-Hale K, Lin E, Tellez C, Deng W, Gopal YN, et al. Integrated molecular and clinical analysis of AKT activation in metastatic melanoma. Clinical Cancer Research. 2009;**15**(24):7538-7546

[63] Niessner H, Forschner A, Klumpp B, Honegger JB, Witte M, Mornemann A, et al. Targeting hyperactivation of the AKT survival pathway to overcome therapy resistance of melanoma brain metastases. Cancer Medicine. 2013;**2**(2):76-85

[64] Hugo W, Shi H, Sun L, Piva M, Song C, Kong X, et al. Non-genomic and immune evolution of melanoma acquiring MAPKi resistance. Cell. 2015;**162**(6):1271-1285

[65] Manzano JL, Layos L, Buges C, de los Llanos Gil M, Vila L, Martinez-Balibrea E, et al. Resistant mechanisms to BRAF inhibitors in melanoma. Annals of Translational Medicine. 2016;**4**(12):237

[66] Long GV, Fung C, Menzies AM, Pupo GM, Carlino MS, Hyman J, et al. Increased MAPK reactivation in early resistance to dabrafenib/trametinib combination therapy of BRAF-mutant metastatic melanoma. Nature Communications. 2014;**5**:5694

[67] Rizos H, Menzies AM, Pupo GM, Carlino MS, Fung C, Hyman J, et al. BRAF inhibitor resistance mechanisms in metastatic melanoma: Spectrum and clinical impact. Clinical Cancer Research. 2014;**20**(7):1965-1977

[68] Ebert PJR, Cheung J, Yang Y, McNamara E, Hong R, Moskalenko M, et al. MAP kinase inhibition promotes T cell and anti-tumor activity in combination with PD-L1 checkpoint blockade. Immunity. 2016;**44**(3):609-621

[69] Hu-Lieskovan S, Mok S, Homet Moreno B, Tsoi J, Robert L, Goedert L, et al. Improved antitumor activity of immunotherapy with BRAF and MEK inhibitors in BRAF(V600E) melanoma. Science Translational Medicine. 2015;**7**:279ra41

[70] Ribas A, Butler M, Lutzky J, Lawrence DP, Robert C, Miller W, et al. Phase I study combining anti-PD-L1 (MEDI4736) with BRAF (dabrafenib) and/or MEK (trametinib) inhibitors in advanced melanoma. Journal of Clinical Oncology. 2015;**33**:3003

[71] Hwu P, Hamid O, Gonzalez R, Infante JR, Patel MR, Hodi FS, et al. Preliminary safety and clinical activity of atezolizumab combined with cobimetinib and vemurafenib in BRAF V600-mutant metastatic melanoma. Annals of Oncology. 2016;**27**(6):1109PD

[72] Sullivan RJ, Gonzalez R, Lewis KD, Hamid O, Infante JR, Patel MR, et al. Atezolizumab (A) + cobimetinib (C) + vemurafenib (V) in BRAFV600-mutant metastatic melanoma (mel): Updated safety and clinical activity. Journal of Clinical Oncology. 2017;**35**(15):3063

[73] Ribas A, Hodi S, Lawrence DP, Atkinson V, Starodub A, Carlino MS, et al. Pembrolizumab (pembro) in combination with dabrafenib (D) and trametinib (T) for BRAF-mutant advanced melanoma: Phase 1 KEYNOTE-022 study. Journal of Clinical Oncology. 2016;**34**(15):3014

[74] Ascierto PA, Ferrucci PF, Stephens R, Del Vecchio M, Atkinson V, Schmidt H, et al. KEYNOTE-022 Part 3: Phase 2 randomized study of 1L dabrafenib (D) and trametinib (T) plus pembrolizumab (pembro) or placebo (PBO) for BRAF-mutant advanced melanoma. Annals of Oncology. 2018;**29**(8):mdy289

Chapter 2

Atypical Protein Kinase Cs in Melanoma Progression

Wishrawana S. Ratnayake, Christopher A. Apostolatos and Mildred Acevedo-Duncan

Abstract

Melanoma is one of the fastest growing types of cancer worldwide in terms of incidence. To date, reports show over 92,000 new cases in the United States in 2018. Previously, we introduced protein kinase C-iota (PKC-ι) as an oncogene in melanoma. PKC-ι promotes survival and cancer progression along with PKC-zeta(ζ). In addition, we reported that PKC-ι induced metastasis of melanoma cells by increasing Vimentin dynamics. Our previous results showed that PKC-ι inhibition downregulated epithelial-mesenchymal transition (EMT), while inducing apoptosis. In this chapter, we summarized these findings which were based on the *in-vitro* applications of five specific atypical PKC (aPKC) inhibitors. In addition, the underlying mechanisms of the transcriptional regulation of PRKCI gene expression in melanoma is also discussed. Results demonstrated that c-Jun promotes PRKCI expression along with Interleukin (IL)-6/8. Furthermore, forkhead box protein O1 (FOXO1) acts as a downregulator of PRKCI expression upon stimulation of IL-17E and intercellular adhesion molecule 1 (ICAM-1) in melanoma cells. Overall, the chapter summarizes the importance of PKC-ι/ζ in the progression of melanoma and discusses the cellular signaling pathways that are altered upon inhibitor applications. Finally, we established that aPKCs are effective novel biomarkers for use in the design of novel targeted therapeutics for melanoma.

Keywords: PKC-iota (ι), PKC-zeta (ζ), metastasis, FOXO1, c-Jun

1. Introduction

The protein kinase C (PKC) is a family of Ser/Thr kinases which are involved in transmembrane signal transduction pathways triggered by various extra and intracellular stimuli [1]. Over time, more information has become available since the 1st discovery of PKCs in 1970s. Activation of PKCs may depend on calcium ions and cofactors like the lipid metabolite diacylglycerol (DAG) and phosphatidylserine (PS) [2, 3]. The PKC family consists of fifteen isozymes which are grouped into three on the basis of their co-factor requirements [4, 5]. First group is the conventional PKCs (cPKC) which includes the isoforms alpha (α), beta I (βI), beta II (βII) and gamma (γ) and they require calcium ions, DAG and phospholipids for the activation. Second group is the novel PKCs (nPKC) and it includes delta (δ), epsilon (ε), eta (η) and theta (θ). These are calcium ion independent but dependent on DAG and phospholipids. The aPKC isozymes are the third group, which are independent of Calcium and DAG for their activation. PKC-ζ and PKC-ι in humans (lambda (λ) is the mouse homologs of iota) are the three aPKCs. Protein kinase D, mu (μ) and some PKC-related kinases (PRK1, PRK2 and PRK3), known as PKN are also considered as PKCs [6].

PKCs have extremely conserved carboxyl-terminal catalytic domain (kinase domain) and PKC isozymes differ from each other on the basis of their amino-terminal (N-terminal) regulatory domain. The N-terminal domain is very important for secondary messenger binding, recruiting the enzyme to the membrane and protein-protein interactions [2]. The pseudosubstrate (PS) domain is located at the N-terminal. PS has a peptide-sequence similar to that of a substrate but lacks alanine in the phosphoacceptor position. In the inactive form of PKCs, the PS prevents complete activation of PKC by blocking the substrate binding pocket [7]. The PS is released upon activation [8, 9]. The activation of PKCs typically involves a cascade of three coordinated phosphorylation events [10, 11]. First, phosphorylation takes place at the activation loop triggered by phosphoinositide-dependent kinase-1 (PDK-1) [12–14]. This initiates a chain reaction that involves autophosphorylation at the turn motif that further stimulates the autophosphorylation at hydrophobic motif of N-terminal [13]. The autophosphorylation at hydrophobic motif is the third and concluding step of the activation.

Atypical PKCs contains two structurally and functionally distinct isozymes in human, PKC-ı and PKC-ζ. The amino acid sequences in both PKC-ı and PKC-ζ are very similar to each other [15, 16]. PKC-ı is encoded by the PRKCI gene and PKC-ζ is encoded by the PRKCZ gene. They are believed to be involved in cell cycle progression, tumorigenesis, cell survival and cell migration of carcinoma cells. Additionally, aPKCs play important roles in insulin-stimulated glucose transport [16, 17]. PKC-ı specifically has a strong influence on cell cycle progression. It is also involved in changing cell polarity during cell division [17]. Lung cancer cell proliferation is highly dependent on the PKC-ı level since it increases tumor cell proliferation by activating the ERK1 pathway [15]. PKC-ı and PKC-ζ are expressed in both transformed and malignant melanoma [18]. Overexpression of PKC-ı plays an important role in the chemoresistance of leukemia [19]. PKC-ı is involved in glioma cell proliferation by regulating by phosphorylation of cyclin-dependent kinase activating kinase/cyclin-dependent kinase 7 pathway [20, 21]. A very important study by Selzer et al., investigated the presence of 11 PKC isoforms in 8 different melanoma metastases, 3 normal melanocyte cell lines and 3 spontaneously transformed melanocytes along with several melanoma tumor samples. PKC-ζ and PKC-ı

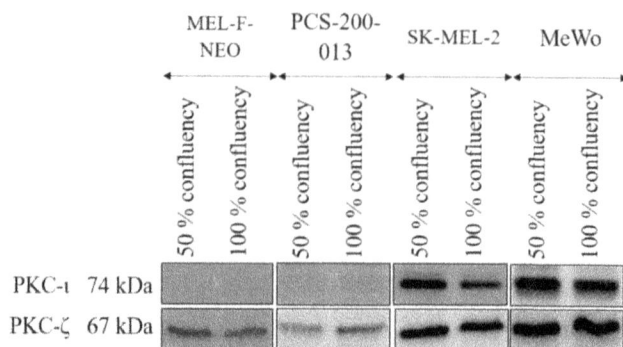

Figure 1.
aPKC expression comparison of normal melanocytes and melanoma cell lines. The expression of PKC-ı and PKC-ζ was reported at approximately 50 and 100% confluency for PCS-200-013 and MEL-F-NEO normal melanocytes against SK-MEL-2 and MeWo metastatic melanoma cells. Western blots were conducted with 50 µg of total proteins loaded in each lane and the complete procedure was adapted from Ratnayake et al. [67].

were found in all transformed melanocytes and melanoma metastases samples in very high levels. PKC-ζ was also found in normal melanocytes in low levels. **Figure 1** demonstrates a comparison of the aPKC expression in two normal melanocyte cell lines (PCS-200-013 and MEL-F-NEO) against two melanoma cell lines (SK-MEL-2 and MeWo) which were used for our studies in Acevedo-Duncan's laboratory at the University of South Florida. As demonstrated in **Figure 1**, normal melanocytes did not show detectable levels of PKC-ι compared to the larger expression observed in SK-MEL-2 and MeWo cell lines. Moreover, PKC-ζ expression was very low in both normal melanocyte cell lines compared to heightened expression in melanoma cells. These results supported the expression patterns demonstrated by patient samples as described in Selzer et al. [18]. All these results indicate a strong relationship between aPKCs and melanoma progression. Here, we discuss our key findings of our recent research on melanoma owing to its relationship with aPKCs in a detailed manner.

2. Atypical PKCs promote cell differentiation, survival of melanoma cells via NF-κB and PI3K/AKT pathways

Nuclear factor kappa-light-chain-enhancer of activated B (NF-κB) and phosphatidylinositol 3-kinase and protein kinase B (PI3K/AKT) pathways are often hyper-activated in many different cancers in order to promote cellular differentiation, growth and survival. Overexpression of aPKCs is often associated with anti-apoptotic effects in many cancers. We have published outcomes of *in-vitro* treatments of aPKC specific inhibitors in which, treatments decreased melanoma cell population markedly compared to normal melanocytes [22–25]. These results confirm that melanoma cellular functions are highly dependent on aPKCs, but normal melanocytes do not depend on aPKCs.

Our recent publications describe the *in-vitro* effects of five aPKC inhibitors on melanoma cell lines compared to normal melanocytes [22, 23]. 2-Acetyl-1, 3-cyclopentanedione (ACPD) and 3,4-diaminonaphthalene-2,7-disulfonic acid (DNDA) are specific to both PKC-ι and PKC-ζ while [4-(5-amino-4-carbamoylimidazol-1-yl)-2,3-dihydroxycyclopentyl] methyl dihydrogen phosphate (ICA-1T) along with its nucleoside analog 5-amino-1-((1R,2S,3S,4R)-2,3-dihydroxy-4-methylcyclopentyl)-1H-imidazole-4-carboxamide (ICA-1S) which are specific to PKC-ι and 8-hydroxy-1,3,6-naphthalenetrisulfonic acid (ζ-Stat) is specific to PKC-ζ. These compounds were identified from the National Cancer Institute/Developmental Therapeutics Program (NCI/DTP) database using molecular docking simulations. "AutoDockTools" and "AutoDock Vina" programs were used for the docking simulation by selecting structural pockets in PKC-ι and PKC-ζ which were compatible with small drug like molecules. Sixteen different pockets were identified on PKC-ι and PKC-ζ structures using "fpocket," a very fast open source protein pocket (cavity) detection system based on Voronoi Tessellation. We confirmed the presence of a potentially druggable allosteric site in the structure of PKC-ι using solved crystal structure of PKC-ι. The pocket located in C-lobe of the kinase domain, is framed by solvent exposed residues of helices αF-αI and the activation segment. PKC-ι inhibitors were predicted to interact with this site with moderate affinity based on molecular docking. Combinations of drugs targeting the ATP binding site and allosteric sites would be expected to more effectively inhibit cancer cell growth [23]. More details about other aPKC inhibitors form different research groups can be found in the latter portion of the chapter.

All five inhibitors were cytostatic to malignant cells rather than cytotoxic. Cells underwent growth arrest before apoptotic stimulation. Regardless, ICA-1S and ICA-1T showed a minor toxicity towards malignant melanoma cells, suggesting that all inhibitors were effective against malignant cells without harming normal cells. This is an indication that melanoma cells heavily rely on aPKCs to remain viable which was observed in some other cancers [19, 20, 26, 27]. These previous reports show that overexpression of aPKCs have an anti-apoptotic effect [15, 19–21, 28, 29]. Our two previous publications on the applications of aPKC specific inhibitors report apoptosis analysis on MeWo and SK-MEL-2 cells. The data confirmed that inhibition of aPKCs lead to induce apoptosis [22, 23]. Increase in Caspase-3, increase in poly ADP ribose polymerase (PARP) cleavage, and a decrease in B-cell lymphoma-2 (Bcl-2) all indicate apoptosis stimulation [30–33]. All five inhibitors have demonstrated similar pattern on these markers. But, increase in Caspase-3 levels is not always a direct indication of inducing the apoptosis due to the tight binding of cleaved Caspase-3 with X-linked inhibitor of apoptosis protein (XIAP). XIAP undergoes auto-ubiquitylation, but this process delays apoptosis until all XIAP is removed [34]. On the other hand, PARP is a known downstream target for Caspase-3, therefore we have also tested direct PARP and cleaved PARP levels upon inhibitor treatments. PARP cleavage increases upon inducing the apoptosis [35]. Bcl-2 inhibits Caspase activity by preventing Cytochrome c release from the mitochondria and/or by binding to the apoptosis-activating factor (APAF-1). In our studies, PKC-ι and PKC-ζ inhibition decreased Bcl-2 levels which depicted an increase in apoptotic activity in both SK-MEL-2 and MeWo cell lines. These data confirms that aPKCs have an anti-apoptotic effect in the tested melanoma cells.

PI3K/AKT mediated NF-κB activation is a major anti-apoptotic pathway, wherein aPKCs play a role in releasing NF-κB complex to translocate to the nucleus and promote cell survival. Win et al. reported that PKC-ζ actively upregulates the activation of NF-κB nuclei translocation thereby inducing cancer cell survival in prostate cancer cells [36, 37]. In addition, PI3K stimulates IκB kinase (IKKα/β) through activation of AKT by phosphorylation at S473 or S463, which ultimately stimulates translocation of NF-κB complex into the nucleus, heightening cell survival [38]. Phosphatase and tensin homolog (PTEN) regulates the levels of PI3K. Phosphorylation at S380 leads to the inactivation of PTEN, thereby increasing the levels of PI3K followed by enhancement in phosphorylated AKT (S473/S463). Our data indicates that inhibition of PKC-ι and PKC-ζ expressively decreased the levels of phosphorylated PTEN and phosphorylated AKT [23]. This specifies that PKC-ζ and PKC-ι may upregulate the PI3K/AKT pathway to induce cellular survival of melanoma cells. Additionally, we tested the levels of NF-κB translocation by separating the nuclear extracts from the cell lysates and found that NF-κB levels in the nuclei decreased upon aPKC inhibition. This suggested that translocation of activated NF-κB into nuclei was blocked as a result of inhibition of aPKCs. Furthermore, we also found that aPKC inhibition increased the levels of inhibitor of kappa B (IκB) while decreasing the levels of phosphorylated IκB (S32) and phosphorylated IKKα/β (S176/180), confirming that both PKC-ι and PKC-ζ play a role in phosphorylation of IKKα/β and IκB: increased levels of IκB therefore remain bound to NF-κB complex and prevent the translocation to the nucleus to promote cell survival (**Figure 2**). As summarized in **Figure 2**, our data also demonstrate the effects of TNF-α stimulation on the expression of aPKCs [23]. TNF-α is a cytokine, involved in the early phase of acute inflammation by activating NF-κB. TNF-α stimulation significantly increased NF-κB levels in both cytosol and nuclei. Increased NF-κB production promotes increases in total and phosphorylated aPKCs and increased the levels of Bcl-2, which enhanced melanoma cell survival. We observed amplified levels of IκB and NF-κB, which together enhanced the phosphorylation of IκB due to the augmented levels of aPKCs [23]. On the other hand, PI3K/AKT signaling can be diminished by inhibiting aPKCs via downregulation of NF-κB. These results confirm that both PKC-ζ and PKC-ι are rooted in cellular survival via NF-κB and PI3K/AKT pathways.

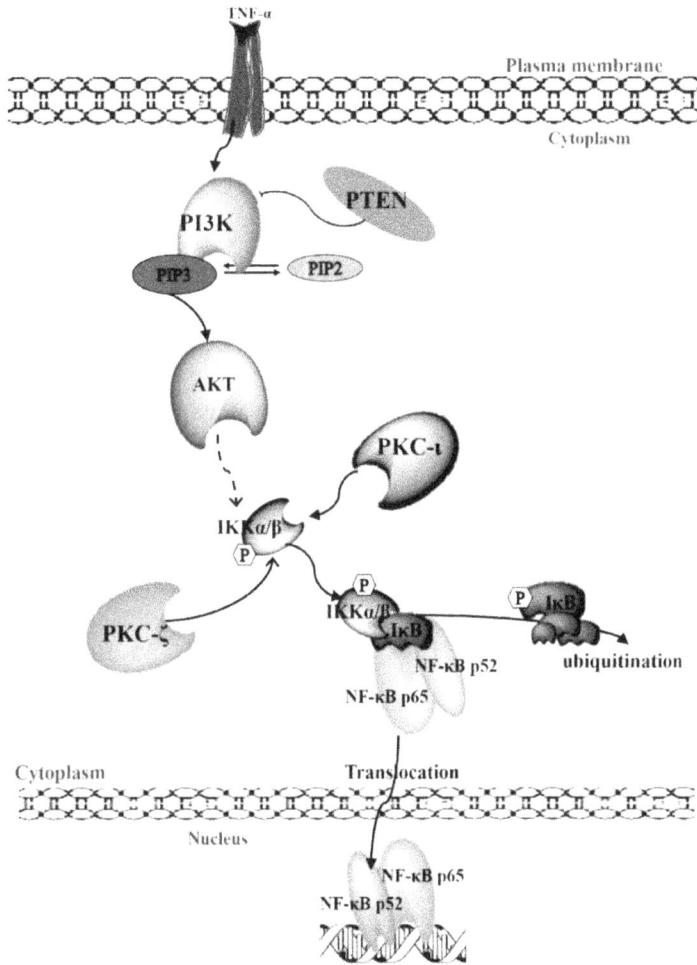

Figure 2.
A schematic summary of the involvement of PKC-ι and PKC-ζ in melanoma progression via NF-κB and PI3K/ AKT pathways. Upon extracellular stimulation with TNF-α, activation of AKT through PIP₃ takes place as a result of inactivation of PTEN. Activated AKT pathway can lead to cell survival, rapid proliferation and differentiation which are critical parts of melanoma progression. AKT could indirectly stimulate NF-κB pathway along with PKC-ι and PKC-ζ in which they play a stimulatory role on IKK-α/β in order to promote the releasing the NF-κB complex from IκB to translocate into nucleus.

3. PKC-ι promotes metastasis by promoting epithelial-mesenchymal transition (EMT) and activating Vimentin

Throughout EMT, epithelial cells lose apical-basal polarity, remodel the extra cellular matrix (ECM), rearrange the cytoskeleton, drive changes in signaling programs that control the cell shape maintenance and adapt gene expression to obtain mesenchymal phenotype, which is invasive and increases individual cell motility [39]. EMT's key features comprise downregulation of E-cadherin to destabilize tight junctions between cells and upregulation of genes such as Vimentin that may assist mesenchymal phenotype.

Vimentin is a very important structural protein which belongs to the family of type III intermediate filament proteins. Intermediate filaments (IFs) make up a vast network of interconnecting proteins between the plasma membrane and the nuclear envelope and convey molecular and mechanical information between the cell surface and the nucleus. IF protein expression is cell type and tissue specific. Mesenchymal cells, fibroblasts, lymphocytes and most types of tumor cells express Vimentin [40, 41]. Vimentin is essential for organizing microfilament systems, changing cell polarity, and thereby changing cellular motility. Moreover, increased Vimentin expression during EMT is a hallmark of metastasis which plays a very important role in gaining rear-to-front polarity for transforming epithelial cells. In addition to EMT, Vimentin expression is observed in cell mechanisms involved in cellular development, immune response and wound healing [22, 23, 42].

Vimentin is activated via phosphorylation. Various kinases such as; RhoA kinase, protein kinase A, PKC, Ca^{2+}/calmodulin-dependent protein kinase II (CaM kinase II), cyclin-dependent kinase 1 (CDK1), RAC-alpha serine/threonine-protein kinase (AKT1) and RAF proto-oncogene serine/threonine-protein kinases (Raf-1-associated kinases) have been shown to play a role in regulation of Vimentin via phosphorylation. Studies show that amino acid sites S6, S7, S8, S33, S38 (same as S39 since some literature use M as the starting amino acid of Vimentin), S55 (or S56), S71, S72, and S82 (S83) amongst others, serve as specific phosphorylation sites on the head region of Vimentin [41, 43–50].

Our previous reports demonstrated the effects of aPKC inhibition on melanoma cell migration and invasion [22, 23]. Migration and invasion studies in cancer research are very important because the main cause of death in cancer patients is related to metastatic progression. For cancer cells to spread and distribute through-out the body, they must migrate and invade through ECM, undergo intravasation into blood stream and extravasation to form distant tumors [51]. ACPD and DNDA treated samples demonstrated a reduction of melanoma motility but it was not conclusive which aPKC is responsible for upregulating metastasis, since both ACPD and DNDA inhibit PKC-ι and PKC-ζ [22]. This was solved using specific PKC-ι inhibitors (ICA-1S and ICA-1T) and a PKC-ζ specific inhibitor ζ-Stat. Migration and invasion were markedly reduced for samples treated with ICA-1T and ICA-1S compared to ζ-Stat treated samples, suggesting that PKC-ι inhibition significantly diminishes melanoma cell migration and invasion suggesting that only PKC-ι is involved in EMT in melanoma [23]. aPKC/Par6 signaling is known to stimulate EMT upon activation of TGF-β receptors in lung cancer cells. TGF-β activated aPKC/Par6 stimulates degradation of RhoA which leads to the depolymerization of filamentous actin (F-actin) and loss of epithelial structural integrity resulting a reduction in cell-cell adhesion [52]. RhoA is a GTPase, which promotes actin stress fiber formation thereby maintains cell integrity. Furthermore, TGFβ upregulates Zinc finger protein SNAI1 (SNAIL1) and Paired related homeobox-1 (PRRX1) transcription factors that drive genetic reprogramming to facilitate EMT [53]. Cells lose E-cadherin while gaining Vimentin during this process. We have recently reported that inhibition of PKC-ι using ICA-1T and ICA-1S significantly increased the levels of E-cadherin and RhoA while decreasing total and phosphorylated Vimentin (S39) and Par6. None of these protein levels were significantly changed as a result of PKC-ζ inhibition. We also reported that TGFβ treatments increased the expression of PKC-ι, Vimentin, phosphorylated Vimentin and Par6 while decreas-ing E-cadherin and RhoA [23]. These results confirmed the involvement of PKC-ι in EMT stimulation. Immunoprecipitation of PKC-ι confirmed a strong association with Par6 in both melanoma cells which was confirmed with reverse-immunopre-cipitation of Par6. Previously published reports state that both aPKCs associate with Par6 and phosphorylate at S345 [54]. Interestingly, only PKC-ι showed an associa-tion with Par6, which confirmed that PKC-ι is a major activator of EMT in mela-noma. In addition, immunoprecipitation of PKC-ι and Vimentin strongly confirmed an association between PKC-ι and Vimentin [22]. *si*RNA knockdown of PKC-ι and

PKC-ζ, immunofluorescent staining and real time quantitative polymerase chain reaction (RT-qPCR) techniques were also used to study the association of Vimentin with PKC-ι. Our immunofluorescence staining revealed that the shape of melanoma cells significantly changed upon inhibition of PKC-ι. Both Vimentin and PKC-ι levels were relatively low in ICA-1T treated cells in comparison to their respective controls. In addition, invasive characteristics such as formation of lamellipodia, filopodia and invadopodia were distinctively visible in both controls, though they were not apparent in PKC-ι inhibited cells. Reduction of nuclei volume and cell size, also confirmed the growth retardation we observed in melanoma cells upon aPKC inhibitor treatments that had resulted in lesser growth in treated cells. As observed in qPCR experiments, treatments with PKC-ι specific inhibitors ICA-1T and ICA-1S, depicted a corresponding downregulation of PKC-ι suggested that PKC-ι plays a role in its own regulation [23]. This is further discussed in the next topic in Part 4.

Phosphorylation of Vimentin at S39 is required for its activation and inhibition of PKC-ι diminishes this activation process. The reduced levels of total Vimentin observed in Western blots for ICA-1T and ICA-1S treated cells indicate that without PKC-ι, unphosphorylated Vimentin undergoes rapid degradation. In addition to activating Vimentin, PKC-ι appears to play a role in regulating Vimentin expression in some carcinoma cells [55].

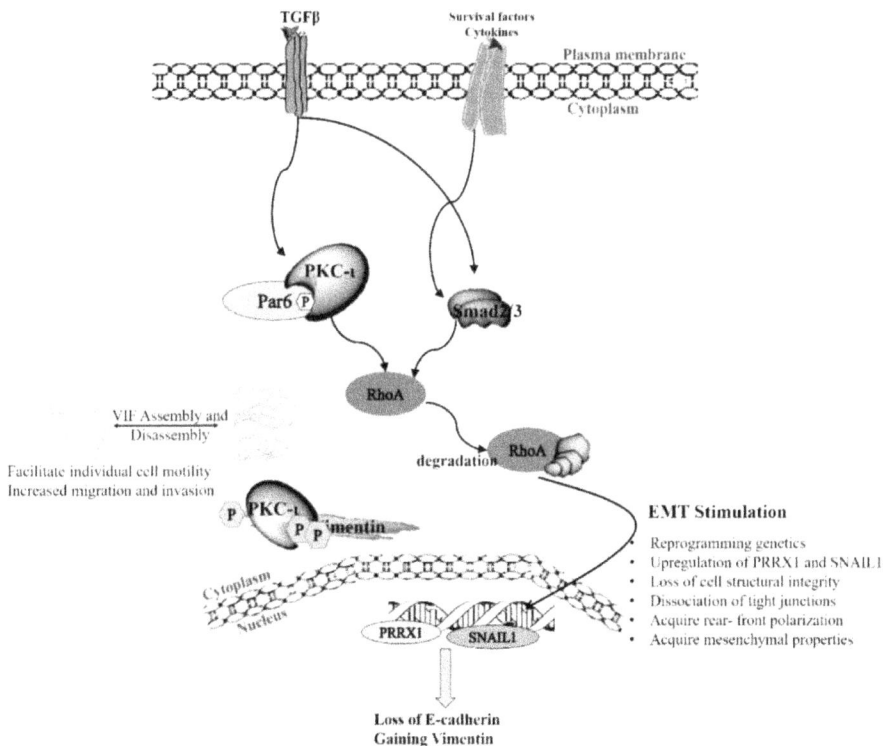

Figure 3.
A schematic summary of the involvement of PKC-ι in melanoma progression via activation of EMT and Vimentin signaling. Upon extracellular stimulation with TGFβ, PKC-ι associates and activates Par6, which stimulates the degradation of RhoA thereby upregulates EMT. SNAIL1 and PRRX1 are two very important transcription factors and they drive EMT process by upregulating Vimentin while downregulating E-cadherin. PKC-ι activates Vimentin by phosphorylation and this initiates disassembly of VIF and facilitates cellular motility. During this process, cadherin junctions are disrupted as a result of loss of E-cadherin and β-catenin is translocated to nucleus to upregulate the production of facilitating proteins such as CD44 which further stimulate migration and EMT. Activated Vimentin changes cell polarity to maintain the mesenchymal phenotype of melanoma cells in-vitro.

As summarized in **Figure 3**, based on our published reports, we believe that TGFβ stimulated PKC-ι/Par6/RhoA and Smad2/3 pathways to induce EMT in melanoma through transcriptional activities of SNAIL1 and PRRX1. Vimentin and PKC-ι activation are upregulated simultaneously to facilitate EMT in melanoma. PKC-ι activated Vimentin thereby regulates the dynamic changes in melanoma metastasis. Our results further confirms that PKC-ι inhibition using specific inhibitors such as ICA-1T and ICA-1S, not only reduce melanoma cell survival but also negatively affects the melanoma metastatic progression by downregulating EMT. Taken together, this novel concept can be used to develop more specific effective therapeutics for melanoma patients based on PKC-ι. PKC-ι can be used as a novel biomarker to mitigate melanoma metastasis using specific inhibitors.

4. Self-regulation of PKC-ι is a crucial mechanism making PKC-ι an important novel target in melanoma anti-cancer therapeutics

In our previous study, we identified PKC-ι as a major component responsible for inducing cell growth, differentiation, survival and EMT promotion in melanoma, as a result of PKC-ι specific inhibitor applications [22, 23]. In addition to these findings, we noted that the inhibition of PKC-ι leads to a decrease in its own expression of PRKCI gene. This indicates that PKC-ι plays a role in its expression in melanoma. The PRKCI gene is located on chromosome 3 (3q26.2), a region identified as an amplicon [56]. Our latest published results describe the transcriptional regulation of PRKCI with an insight view of cell signaling crosstalk in melanoma cells. FOXO1 and c-Jun were identified as possible transcription factors that can bind to the PRKCI promoter region through PROMO and Genomatix Matinspector. These two transcription factors (TFs) were systematically silenced to analyze the downstream effect on PKC-ι expression.

c-Jun is the first discovered oncogenic TF that is associated with metastatic breast cancer, non-small cell lung cancer and several other types of cancer [57–59]. We found a positive correlation between c-Jun with PKC-ι expression. Phosphorylation at S63 and S73 by JNKs (c-Jun N-terminal kinases) activates c-Jun, thereby increasing c-Jun targeted gene transcription. c-Jun stimulates the oncogenic transformation of 'ras' and 'fos' in several type of cancers [60]. FOXO1 is a well-known tumor suppressor and we found it suppresses the expression of oncogenic PKC-ι. FOXO1 also plays a key role in gluconeogenesis, insulin signaling and adipogenesis. AKT is known to deactivate FOXO1 by phosphorylating FOXO1 at T24, which drives FOXO1 nuclear exclusion, leading to ubiquitination [61, 62]. Therefore, the phosphorylation of FOXO1 is an indication of its downregulation. FOXO1 plays a crucial regulatory role in both the intrinsic and extrinsic pathways of apoptosis in many types of cancers, demonstrating an association between FOXO dysregulation and cancer progression [63, 64]. Additionally, upregulation of FOXO1 inhibits cancer cell proliferation, migration and tumorigenesis [65]. Notably, FOXO1 can also be downregulated by ERK1/2 and PKC-ι, in addition to AKT [66]. In our most recent study, we demonstrated that, due to PKC-ι inhibition, the availability of active phosphorylated PKC-ι decreases, making it ineffective at deactivating FOXO1 through phosphorylation at T24. Importantly, this is the first showing direct involvement of PKC-ι in its own expression regulation and PKC-ι inhibition that leads to continuous upregulation of FOXO1 [67].

As we discussed earlier in Part 2, our previous data showed that PKC-ι inhibition significantly downregulated the PI3K/AKT1 pathway, thereby suppressing the activation of AKT [22, 23]. Downregulation of NF-κB due to PKC-ι inhibition, result in downregulation of AKT. Our latest data shows that it increases total FOXO1 level,

while reducing its phosphorylated levels [67]. This confirms that NF-κB downregulation upregulates FOXO1 activity as a result of PKC-ι specific inhibition. Elevated
FOXO1 negatively influenced PKC-ι expression and phosphorylation at T555. This
further confirms our previous observations with PKC-ι inhibition with ICA-1T and
ICA-1S, where total PKC-ι, phosphorylated PKC-ι, NF-κB activation and activated
AKT (S473) were significantly reduced [23]. These results could be due to the tight
regulation of PKC-ι expression by FOXO1, which retards PRKCI from transcription. Such results confirmed that FOXO1 is a major regulator which suppresses the
expression of PRKCI. Interestingly, c-Jun and phosphorylated c-Jun (S63) levels
were not significantly altered as a result of NF-κB siRNA knockdown. This suggests
that NF-κB diminution does not affect PKC-ι expression over c-Jun. Instead, c-Jun is
known to protect cancer cells from apoptosis by cooperating with NF-κB signaling
to facilitate survival upon TNF-α stimulation [68]. These overall effects have been
summarized in **Figure 4**. We have previously shown how TNF-α upregulates NF-κB
and AKT pathways along with PKC-ι expression in these two melanoma cell lines

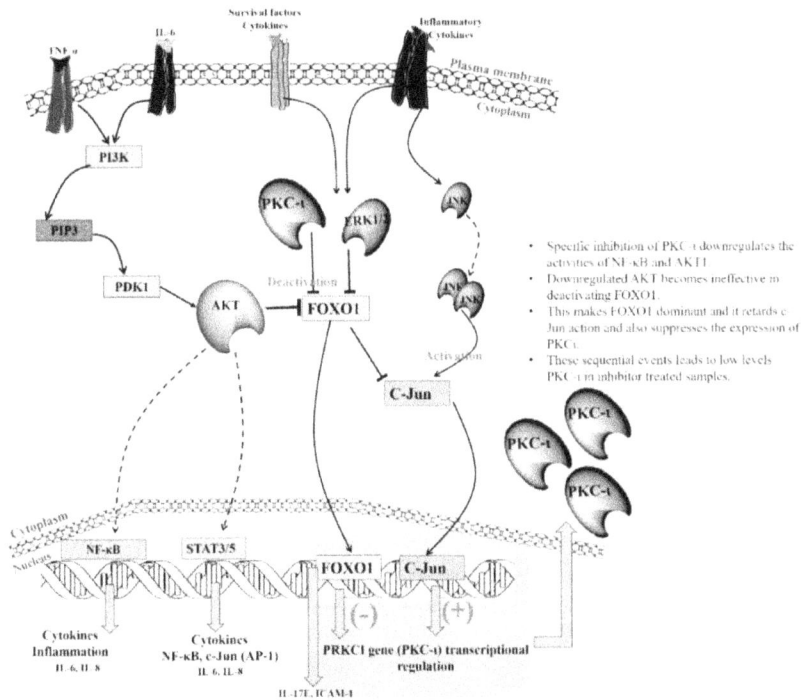

Figure 4.
*A schematic summary of the regulation of the expression of PKC-ι in melanoma. This model depicts the
interactions between NF-κB, PI3K/AKT/FOXO1, JNK/c-Jun and STAT3/5 signaling pathways during the
PKC-ι regulation. PKC-ι plays an important role in the regulation of its own expression in an intricate
signaling web through c-Jun and FOXO1. PKC-ι is overexpressed in melanoma cells due to elevated
transcriptional activity of c-Jun with the aid of PI3K/AKT, NF-κB, STAT3/5 signaling. The specific inhibition
of PKC-ι initiates a disruption to rapid PKC-ι expression cycle in melanoma where the reduced activity
of PKC-ι downregulates the NF-κB pathway and its transcriptional activity, which in turn diminishes the
expression of IL-6/8. As a result of this AKT activity reduction, FOXO1 gets upregulated. FOXO1 turns out
to be the most important TF regulating PKC-ι expression after the disruption initiated as a result of PKC-ι
inhibition. Dominant FOXO1 negatively regulates the expression of PKC-ι and also diminishes the JNK activity
to retard its activation of c-Jun. we found c-Jun as the transcription component which upregulates PKC-ι
expression. The downregulation of IL-6 and IL-8 expression leads to the lessened STAT3/5 signaling, which
causes c-Jun transcriptional reduction. This whole process continues and leads to the further downregulation of
NF-κB, AKT and JNK/c-Jun while upregulating FOXO1, which leads to the continuation of the attenuation of
PKC-ι expression. As a result, the total PKC-ι level decreases in melanoma cells.*

[23]. However, the data from the current study suggest that the TNF-α downstream target is mainly FOXO1, where it 'switches off' through the phosphorylation of elevated AKT. The inhibition of PKC-ι diminishes this AKT activation, thereby upregulating FOXO1 activity [67].

On the other hand, *si*RNA treatments for of c-Jun and FOXO1 revealed that c-Jun also plays a role in PKC-ι expression, apart from FOXO1. Enzyme-linked immunosorbent assay (ELISA) experiments were conducted to investigate cell signaling crosstalks. These findings demonstrated links between PKC-ι expression with the cytokines, interleukin (IL)-6, IL-8, IL-17E and ICAM-1, along with some other key cellular signaling points. Phosphorylation at S536 on the NF-κB p65 transactivation domain is an indication of dimerization of NF-κB subunits. ELISA results revealed a more than two fold increase of NF-κB p65 (S536) in PKC-ι inhibited samples. According to Ratnayake et al., PKC-ι inhibition downregulates NF-κB translocation to the nucleus therefore phospho-NF-κB levels increase in order to diminish the effect of PKC-ι inhibition. However, elevated FOXO1 does not allow NF-κB to annex the control since it is missing the essential assistance needed from PKC-ι due to its inhibition from ICA-1T and ICA-1S inhibitors [67] (**Figure 4**). Abnormal STAT3/5 activity has been shown to be connected to multiple types of cancer [69–72]. Cytokines such as IL-6 and IL-5, upregulate STAT signaling, thereby induces cell survival in many types of cancer [69, 70, 73]. Importantly, upregulated STAT3 increases the transcription of c-Jun [69, 74]. Our ELISA results indicated that STAT3 and STAT5 activities were retarded due to PKC-ι inhibition, signifying c-Jun diminution. Hornsveld et al., and few other reports have provided connections between the JNK pathway and FOXO1, explaining its tumor suppressing features by weakening JNK activity [75, 76]. However, JNK activates c-Jun. Our latest Western blot and real time qPCR analysis demonstrated that c-Jun depletion lessened PKC-ι expression, which suggested that c-Jun acts as an activator of PKC-ι expression. This confirms that both FOXO1 and c-Jun are involved in regulating PKC-ι expression. The results suggest that FOXO1 plays a major role over c-Jun only upon PKC-ι inhibition, possibly through multiple mechanisms, such as the reduction of JNK signaling, retarding PKC-ι expression and cell cycle arrest. FOXO1 induces cell cycle arrest by promoting the transcription of cell cycle kinase inhibitors or cyclin-dependent kinase inhibitor (CKI). p21 and p27 are two well-known downstream CKIs induced by FOXOs [66, 75]. Especially, FOXO1 is also believed to induce anoikis, which is apoptosis that occurs when cells detach from the extracellular matrix. Our ELISA results revealed significantly higher levels of p21 in PKC-ι inhibited cells, suggesting that the inhibition of PKC-ι induces cell cycle arrest through FOXO1 [67]. This also explains why apoptosis was stimulated in melanoma cells as a result of inhibition of PKC-ι in addition to downregulation of PI3K/AKT and NF-κB pathways. Overall, FOXO1 is very important in enhancing anti-tumor activities upon PKC-ι inhibition and it plays the central role of oncogenic PKC-ι depletion.

The next three paragraphs focus on more details concerning cytokine expression changes observed as a result of PKC-ι inhibition [67]. IL-6, IL-8, IL-17E and ICAM-1 expression were significantly altered in melanoma cells upon PKC-ι knockdown [67]. As shown by the results of both Western blot and RT-qPCR analyses, the protein levels of IL-6 and IL-8 (as well as their mRNA levels) decreased, while the levels of IL-17E and ICAM-1 increased significantly upon PKC-ι knockdown by *si*RNA [67]. This suggests that c-Jun and FOXO1 driven PKC-ι expression is involved in autocrine signaling. The micro-environment of a tumor, and in particular melanoma, is regularly exposed to numerous inflammatory factors and immune cells. The effect of these factors function to either promote chronic inflammation or engage in antitumor activity [77]. Cytokines are examples of these inflammatory factors; they play an essential role in regulating the tumor microenvironments [78].

They are vital in order to promote or dysregulate tumor progression and metastasis. Chemokine C-X-C motif ligand-1 (CXCL)-1, CXCL-12, IL-18, CXCL-10, IL-6 and IL-8 are known to promote cancer metastasis. Interestingly, CXCL-1, CXCL-10, CXCL-12 and IL-18 levels were not significantly altered due to PKC-ι depletion in melanoma cells.

IL-6 contributes to the degradation of IκB-α, leading to the upregulation of NF-κB translocation. We have previously discussed that PKC-ι stimulates NF-κB translocation through IκB-α degradation [23]. The translocation of NF-κB to the nucleus induces cell survival through the transcription of various survival factors as well as other pro-survival cytokines [69, 73, 79]. IL-8 plays a role in regulating polymorphonuclear neutrophil mobilization. In melanoma, IL-8 has been attributed to extravasation, a key step in metastasis. Studies have shown that the expression of IL-8 in melanoma is regulated via NF-κB. When NF-κB is translocated to the nucleus, IL-8 expression increases, leading to the promotion of a more favorable microenvironment for metastasis [80, 81]. Our results indicated that both IL-6 and IL-8 expression levels decreased upon diminution of PKC-ι [67].

Some cytokines promote anti-tumor activity by exploiting an immune response. ICAM-1 plays a key role in the immune response, including antigen recognition and lymphocyte activation [82, 83]. ICAM-1 is known for the inhibition of tumor progression through the inhibition of the PI3K/AKT pathway. Tumor cells are exposed to cytotoxic T-lymphocytes as a result of ICAM-1 [83]. According to ovarian cancer clinical data, inhibition of ICAM-1 expression is associated with an increased risk of metastasis for the patients within the first 5 years from the point of diagnosis [82, 83]. IL-17E (IL-25) is another anti-tumor cytokine belongs to a family of cytokines known as IL-17. Treatment with recombinant active IL-17E has been shown to decrease tumor growth of melanoma and pancreatic cancer [84, 85]. The upregulation of IL-17E is linked to the increased expression of TH17 cells. T cells, such as TH17 have been implicated in the inhibition of tumor-infiltrating effector T cells. The exact mechanism of IL-17E function in the anti-tumor effect has not been studied well enough [86]. Particularly, our most recent results indicated that ICAM-1 and IL-17E protein levels and mRNA expression increased upon PKC-ι knockdown by *si*RNA [67]. This strongly supports that anti-tumor signaling is upregulated upon the knockdown or inhibition of oncogenic PKC-ι via an autocrine manner through IL-17E and ICAM-1. Moreover, the results suggest that IL-17E and ICAM-1 play an important down-regulatory role in the regulation of PKC-ι expression along with FOXO1, opposite to IL-6/8 assisted c-Jun [67].

In conclusion, based on the published results from Acevedo-Duncan's laboratory and other available information, it is suggested that PKC-ι itself plays an important role in its expression in a complex signaling web through the transcriptional activation/deactivation of c-Jun and FOXO1. The retarded activity of PKC-ι due to application of specific inhibitors such as ICA-1S and ICA-1T, causes a down-regulation of the NF-κB pathway and its transcriptional activity, which reduces the expression/production of IL-6 and IL-8. In addition, as a result, the activity of AKT decreases, upregulation of FOXO1 activity takes place. FOXO1 is the most important TF regulating PKC-ι expression and IL-17E and ICAM-1 cytokines seem to play a stimulatory role for FOXO1 to attenuate PKC-ι. FOXO1 negatively regulates the expression of PKC-ι, diminishing JNK activity which leads to retard c-Jun activation. IL-6 and IL-8 expression are downregulated via PKC-ι-mediated NF-κB transcriptional activity reduction. IL-6/8 attenuation leads to STAT3/5 signaling downregulation, further reducing c-Jun expression. This whole process continues and leads to the further downregulation of NF-κB, c-Jun and upregulation of FOXO1, which leads to the continuation of the depletion of PKC-ι expression. As a result of this sequence of events, the total PKC-ι level decreases in melanoma cells, which initiated as a result of PKC-ι inhibition using specific inhibitors. These results indicate that PKC-ι is being regulated in a rather complex manner, which involves itself as a key component. PKC-ι specific inhibition using ICA-1S and ICA-1T leads to a decrease in its own production, and during this process, PKC-ι inhibition also triggers multiple anti-tumor/pro-apoptotic signaling. This makes PKC-ι one of the central key points of interest to specifically target and diminish as a means of treating melanoma. The results also strongly suggest that PKC-ι is a prime novel biomarker that can be targeted to design and develop personalized and targeted therapeutics for melanoma.

5. State of atypical PKC inhibitors

We have discussed the effects of five aPKC specific inhibitors throughout this chapter. The structures of these compounds are shown in **Figure 5**.

Atypical PKCs were first considered as a novel therapeutic target by Stallings-Mann et al. in 2006. They screened aurothiomalate as a potent inhibitor of the interaction between PB1 domain of PKC-ι and Par6 [87]. Half maximal inhibitory concentration (IC50) of aurothiomalate ranged from 300 nM to 100 μM and indicated that some cell lines are insensitive (i.e. H460 and A549 lung cancer cells) to the inhibitor [87].

Blázquez et al. tested calphostin C and chelerythrine against West Nile virus (WNV) which significantly inhibit WNV multiplication in cell culture without affecting cell viability. They report that PKCs have also been implicated in different steps during viral replication. Calphostin C and chelerythrine two wide range PKC inhibitors that target all three PKC classes. Results indicate that atypical PKCs are involved in WNV multiplication process which can be effectively retard using said inhibitors [88].

Kim et al. reported the application of Echinochrome A as an inducer of cardio-myocyte differentiation from mouse embryonic stem cells. Echinochrome A was

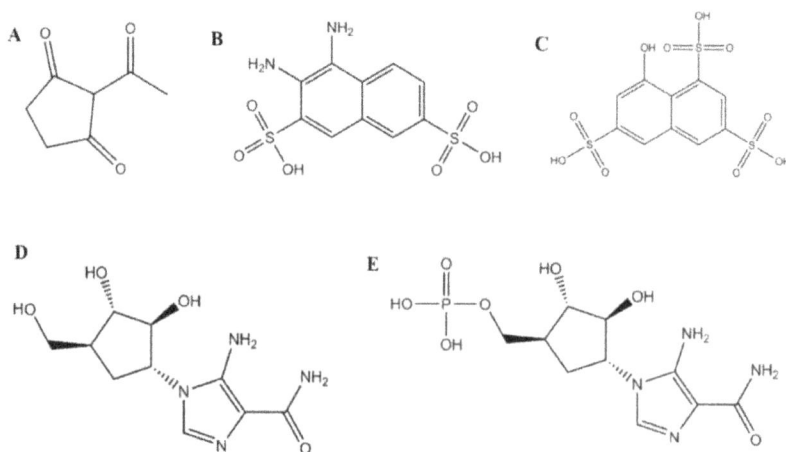

Figure 5.
Structures of the aPKC specific inhibitors (ACPD, DNDA, ζ-Stat, ICA-1S and ICA-1T). chemical structures of ACPD (a) and DNDA are specific to both PKC-ι and PKC-ζ, ζ-Stat (C) is specific to PKC-ζ while ICA-1S (D) and ICA-1T (E) are specific to PKC-ι. molecular weights (MW) of ACPD (140.14 g/mol), DNDA (318.32 g/mol), ζ-Stat (MW = 384.34 g/mol), ICA-1S (MW = 256.26 g/mol) and ICA-1T (MW = 336.24 g/mol), respectively.

extracted from sea urchins. They investigated the potential use of Echinochrome A as an aPKC specific inhibitor and found that IC_{50} for PKC-ι is 107 μM under *in-vitro* kinase assay conditions. Molecular docking simulation results suggested a direct binding of Echinochrome A with PKC-ι [89].

An important study by Kwiatkowski et al. identified an azaindole-based scaffold for the development of more potent and specific PKC-ι inhibitors. They described fragmented based approach an introduced a new class of potential aPKC inhibitors based on azaindole [90].

Acknowledgements

The authors acknowledge the generous financial contributions from the Frederick H. Leonhardt Foundation, David Tanner Foundation, Bradley Zankel Foundation, Inc., Kyrias Foundation, Brotman Foundation of California, Baker Hughes Foundation, Irving S. Cooper Family Foundation, and the Creag Foundation.

Conflict of interests

The authors declare that they have no competing interests.

Author details

Wishrawana S. Ratnayake, Christopher A. Apostolatos
and Mildred Acevedo-Duncan*
Department of Chemistry, University of South Florida, Tampa, FL, USA

*Address all correspondence to: macevedo@usf.edu

IntechOpen

References

[1] Kishimoto A, Takai Y, Mori T, Kikkawa U, Nishizuka Y. Activation of calcium and phospholipid-dependent protein kinase by diacylglycerol, its possible relation to phosphatidylinositol turnover. The Journal of Biological Chemistry. 1980;**255**:2273-2276

[2] Newton AC. Protein kinase C: Structure, function, and regulation. The Journal of Biological Chemistry. 1995;**270**:28495-28498. DOI: 10.1074/jbc.270.48.28495

[3] Kaibuchi K, Takai Y, Nishizuka Y. Protein kinase C and calcium ion in mitogenic response of macrophage-depleted human peripheral lymphocytes. The Journal of Biological Chemistry. 1985;**260**:1366-1369

[4] Hausser A, Storz P, Hübner S, Braendlin I, Martinez-Moya M, Link G, et al. Protein kinase C μ selectively activates the mitogen-activated protein kinase (MAPK) p42 pathway. FEBS Letters. 2001;**492**:39-44. DOI: 10.1016/S0014-5793(01)02219-0

[5] Webb BLJ, Hirst SJ, Giembycz MA. Protein kinase C isoenzymes: A review of their structure, regulation and role in regulating airways smooth muscle tone and mitogenesis. British Journal of Pharmacology. 2000;**130**:1433-1452. DOI: 10.1038/sj.bjp.0703452

[6] Palmer RH, Ridden J, Parker PJ. Cloning and expression patterns of two members of a novel protein-kinase-C-related kinase family. European Journal of Biochemistry. 1995;**227**:344-351. DOI: 10.1111/j.1432-1033.1995.tb20395.x

[7] House C, Kemp BE. Protein kinase C contains a pseudosubstrate prototope in its regulatory domain. Science. 1987;**238**:1726-1728. DOI: 10.1126/science.3686012

[8] Orr JW, Newton AC. Intrapeptide regulation of protein kinase C. The Journal of Biological Chemistry. 1994;**269**:8383-8387

[9] Orr JW, Keranen LM, Newton AC. Reversible exposure of the pseudosubstrate domain of protein kinase C by phosphatidylserine and diacylglycerol. The Journal of Biological Chemistry. 1992;**267**:15263-15266

[10] Tsutakawa SE, Medzihradszky KF, Flint AJ, Burlingame AL, Koshland DE. Determination of in vivo phosphorylation sites in protein kinase C. The Journal of Biological Chemistry. 1995;**270**:26807-26812. DOI: 10.1074/jbc.270.45.26807

[11] Keranen LM, Dutil EM, Newton AC. Protein kinase C is regulated in vivo by three functionally distinct phosphorylations. Current Biology. 1995;**5**:1394-1403. DOI: 10.1016/S0960-9822(95)00277-6

[12] Johnson LN, Noble MEM, Owen DJ. Active and inactive protein kinases: Structural basis for regulation. Cell. 1996;**85**:149-158. DOI: 10.1016/S0092-8674(00)81092-2

[13] Dutil EM, Toker A, Newton AC. Regulation of conventional protein kinase C isozymes by phosphoinositide-dependent kinase 1 (PDK-1). Current Biology. 1998;**8**:1366-1375. DOI: 10.1016/S0960-9822(98)00017-7

[14] Chou MM, Hou W, Johnson J, Graham LK, Lee MH, Chen C-S, et al. Regulation of protein kinase C ζ by PI 3-kinase and PDK-1. Current Biology. 1998;**8**:1069-1078. DOI: 10.1016/S0960-9822(98)70444-0

[15] Regala RP, Weems C, Jamieson L, Khoor A, Edell ES, Lohse CM, et al. Atypical protein kinase C iota is an oncogene in human non-small cell lung

cancer. Cancer Research. 2005;**65**: 8905-8911. DOI: 10.1158/0008-5472. CAN-05-2372

[16] Bandyopadhyay G, Sajan MP, Kanoh Y, Standaert ML, Quon MJ, Lea-Currie R, et al. PKC-zeta mediates insulin effects on glucose transport in cultured preadipocyte-derived human adipocytes. The Journal of Clinical Endocrinology and Metabolism. 2002;**87**:716-723. DOI: 10.1210/jc.87.2.716

[17] Plant PJ, Fawcett JP, Lin DCC, Holdorf AD, Binns K, Kulkarni S, et al. A polarity complex of mPar-6 and atypical PKC binds, phosphorylates and regulates mammalian Lgl. Nature Cell Biology. 2003;**5**:301-308. DOI: 10.1038/ncb948

[18] Selzer E, Okamoto I, Lucas T, Kodym R, Pehamberger H, Jansen B. Protein kinase C isoforms in normal and transformed cells of the melanocytic lineage. Melanoma Research. 2002;**12**:201-209. DOI: 10.1097/00008390-200206000-00003

[19] Murray NR, Fields AP. Atypical protein kinase C ι protects human leukemia cells against drug-induced apoptosis. The Journal of Biological Chemistry. 1997;**272**:27521-27524. DOI: 10.1074/jbc.272.44.27521

[20] Acevedo-Duncan M, Patel R, Whelan S, Bicaku E. Human glioma PKC-iota, and PKC-beta II phosphorylate cyclin-dependent kinase activating kinase during the cell cycle. Cell Proliferation. 2002;**35**:23-36. DOI: 10.1046/j.1365-2184.2002.00220.x

[21] Patel R, Win H, Desai S, Patel K, Matthews JA, Acevedo-Duncan M. Involvement of PKC-iota in glioma proliferation. Cell Proliferation. 2008;**41**:122-135. DOI: 10.1111/j.1365-2184.2007.00506.x

[22] Ratnayake WS, Apostolatos AH, Ostrov DA, Acevedo-Duncan M. Two novel atypical PKC inhibitors; ACPD and DNDA effectively mitigate cell proliferation and epithelial to mesenchymal transition of metastatic melanoma while inducing apoptosis. International Journal of Oncology. 2017;**51**:1370-1382. DOI: 10.3892/ijo.2017.4131

[23] Ratnayake WS, Apostolatos CA, Apostolatos AH, Schutte RJ, Huynh MA, Ostrov DA, et al. Oncogenic PKC-ι activates Vimentin during epithelial-mesenchymal transition in melanoma; a study based on PKC-ι and PKC-ζ specific inhibitors. Cell Adhesion & Migration. 2018;**0**:1-17. DOI: 10.1080/19336918.2018.1471323

[24] Ratnayake WS, Acevedo-Duncan M. AbstractUse of ACPD and ICA-1 as inhibitors of atypical protein kinase C-zeta (ζ) and iota (ι) in metastasized melanoma cells. Cancer Research. 2016;**76**:4569. DOI: 10.1158/1538-7445. AM2016-4569

[25] Ratnayake WS, Acevedo-Duncan M. Abstract 862: Atypical protein kinase c inhibitors can repress epithelial to mesenchymal transition (type III) in malignant melanoma. Cancer Research. 2017;**77**:862. DOI: 10.1158/1538-7445. AM2017-862

[26] Shultz JC, Vu N, Shultz MD, Mba M-UU, Shapiro BA, Chalfant CE. The proto-oncogene PKC iota regulates the alternative splicing of Bcl-x pre-mRNA. Molecular Cancer Research. 2012;**10**:660-669. DOI: 10.1158/1541-7786.MCR-11-0363

[27] do Carmo A, Balca-Silva J, Matias D, Lopes MC. PKC signaling in glioblastoma. Cancer Biology & Therapy. 2013;**14**:287-294. DOI: 10.4161/cbt.23615

[28] Manning G, Whyte DB, Martinez R, Hunter T, Sudarsanam S. The protein kinase complement of the human genome. Science. 2002;**298**:1912. DOI: 10.1126/science.1075762

[29] Koivunen J, Aaltonen V, Peltonen J. Protein kinase C (PKC) family in cancer progression. Cancer Letters. 2006;**235**:1-10. DOI: 10.1016/j.canlet.2005.03.033

[30] Janicke RU, Sprengart ML, Wati MR, Porter AG. Caspase-3 is required for DNA fragmentation and morphological changes associated with apoptosis. The Journal of Biological Chemistry. 1998;**273**:9357-9360. DOI: 10.1074/jbc.273.16.9357

[31] Kroemer G. The proto-oncogene Bcl-2 and its role in regulating apoptosis. Nature Medicine. 1997;**3**: 614-620. DOI: 10.1038/nm0697-614

[32] Watson A, Askew J, Benson R. Poly(adenosine diphosphate ribose) polymerase inhibition prevents necrosis induced by H_2O_2 but not apoptosis. Gastroenterology. 1995;**109**:472-482. DOI: 10.1016/0016-5085(95)90335-6

[33] Soldani C, Poly SAI. (ADP-ribose) polymerase-1 cleavage during apoptosis: An update. Apoptosis. 2002;**7**:321-328. DOI: 10.1023/A:1016119328968

[34] van Raam BJ, Drewniak A, Groenewold V, van den Berg TK, Kuijpers TW. Granulocyte colony-stimulating factor delays neutrophil apoptosis by inhibition of calpains upstream of caspase-3. Blood. 2008;**112**:2046-2054. DOI: 10.1182/blood-2008-04-149575

[35] Cohen GM. Caspases: The executioners of apoptosis. The Biochemical Journal. 1997;**326**:1-16

[36] Win HY, Acevedo-Duncan M. Atypical protein kinase C phosphorylates IKK alpha beta in transformed non-malignant and malignant prostate cell survival. Cancer Letters. 2008;**270**:302-311. DOI: 10.1016/j.canlet.2008.05.023

[37] Apostolatos AH, Ratnayake WS, Win-Piazza H, Apostolatos CA, Smalley T, Kang L, et al. Inhibition of atypical protein kinase C-ι effectively reduces the malignancy of prostate cancer cells by downregulating the NF-κB signaling cascade. International Journal of Oncology. 2018;**53**:1836-1846. DOI: 10.3892/ijo.2018.4542

[38] Scott M, Fujita T, Liou H, Nolan G, Baltimore D. The P65-subunit of Nf-kappa-B regulates I-kappa-B by 2 distinct mechanisms. Genes & Development. 1993;**7**:1266-1276. DOI: 10.1101/gad.7.7a.1266

[39] Lamouille S, Xu J, Derynck R. Molecular mechanisms of epithelial–mesenchymal transition. Nature Reviews. Molecular Cell Biology. 2014;**15**:178-196. DOI: 10.1038/nrm3758

[40] Lai Y-K, Lee W-C, Chen K-D. Vimentin serves as a phosphate sink during the apparent activation of protein kinases by okadaic acid in mammalian cells. Journal of Cellular Biochemistry. 1993;**53**:161-168. DOI: 10.1002/jcb.240530209

[41] Yasui Y, Goto H, Matsui S, Manser E, Lim L, Ki Null N, et al. Protein kinases required for segregation of vimentin filaments in mitotic process. Oncogene. 2001;**20**:2868-2876. DOI: 10.1038/sj.onc.1204407

[42] Snider NT, Omary MB. Post-translational modifications of intermediate filament proteins: Mechanisms and functions. Nature Reviews. Molecular Cell Biology. 2014;**15**:163-177. DOI: 10.1038/nrm3753

[43] Eriksson JE, He T, Trejo-Skalli AV, Härmälä-Braskén A-S, Hellman J, Chou Y-H, et al. Specific in vivo phosphorylation sites determine the assembly dynamics of vimentin intermediate filaments. Journal of Cell Science. 2004;**117**:919-932. DOI: 10.1242/jcs.00906

[44] Ivaska J, Vuoriluoto K, Huovinen T, Izawa I, Inagaki M, Parker PJ. PKCε-mediated phosphorylation of vimentin controls integrin recycling and motility. The EMBO Journal. 2005;**24**:3834-3845. DOI: 10.1038/sj.emboj.7600847

[45] Goto H, Kosako H, Tanabe K, Yanagida M, Sakurai M, Amano M, et al. Phosphorylation of Vimentin by rho-associated kinase at a unique amino-terminal site that is specifically phosphorylated during cytokinesis. The Journal of Biological Chemistry. 1998;**273**:11728-11736. DOI: 10.1074/jbc.273.19.11728

[46] Zhu Q-S, Rosenblatt K, Huang K-L, Lahat G, Brobey R, Bolshakov S, et al. Vimentin is a novel AKT1 target mediating motility and invasion. Oncogene. 2011;**30**:457-470. DOI: 10.1038/onc.2010.421

[47] Cheng T-J, Tseng Y-F, Chang W-M, Chang MD-T, Lai Y-K. Retaining of the assembly capability of vimentin phosphorylated by mitogen-activated protein kinase-activated protein kinase-2. Journal of Cellular Biochemistry. 2003;**89**:589-602. DOI: 10.1002/jcb.10511

[48] Yamaguchi T, Goto H, Yokoyama T, Silljé H, Hanisch A, Uldschmid A, et al. Phosphorylation by Cdk1 induces Plk1-mediated vimentin phosphorylation during mitosis. The Journal of Cell Biology. 2005;**171**:431-436. DOI: 10.1083/jcb.200504091

[49] Li Q-F, Spinelli AM, Wang R, Anfinogenova Y, Singer HA, Tang DD. Critical role of Vimentin phosphorylation at Ser-56 by p21-activated kinase in Vimentin cytoskeleton signaling. The Journal of Biological Chemistry. 2006;**281**:34716-34724. DOI: 10.1074/jbc.M607715200

[50] Tsujimura K, Ogawara M, Takeuchi Y, Imajoh-Ohmi S, Ha MH, Inagaki M. Visualization and function of vimentin phosphorylation

by cdc2 kinase during mitosis. The Journal of Biological Chemistry. 1994;**269**:31097-31106

[51] Justus CR, Leffler N, Ruiz-Echevarria M, Yang LV. In vitro cell migration and invasion assays. Journal of Visualized Experiments. 2014;**88**: e51046. DOI: 10.3791/51046

[52] Gunaratne A, Di Guglielmo GM. Par6 is phosphorylated by aPKC to facilitate EMT. Cell Adhesion & Migration. 2013;**7**:357-361. DOI: 10.4161/cam.25651

[53] Valcourt U, Kowanetz M, Niimi H, Heldin C-H, Moustakas A. TGF-beta and the Smad signaling pathway support transcriptomic reprogramming during epithelial-mesenchymal cell transition. Molecular Biology of the Cell. 2005;**16**:1987-2002. DOI: 10.1091/mbc.E04-08-0658

[54] Nelson WJ. Remodeling epithelial cell organization: Transitions between front–rear and apical–basal polarity. Cold Spring Harbor Perspectives in Biology. 2009;**1**:A000513. DOI: 10.1101/cshperspect.a000513

[55] Inagaki M, Inagaki N, Takahashi T, Takai Y. Phosphorylation-dependent control of structures of intermediate filaments: A novel approach using site- and phosphorylation state-specific antibodies. Journal of Biochemistry. 1997;**121**:407-414

[56] Butler AM, Buzhardt MLS, Erdogan E, Li S, Inman KS, Fields AP, et al. A small molecule inhibitor of atypical protein kinase C signaling inhibits pancreatic cancer cell transformed growth and invasion. Oncotarget. 2015;**6**:15297-15310. DOI: 10.18632/oncotarget.3812

[57] Vogt PK. Fortuitous convergences: The beginnings of JUN. Nature Reviews. Cancer. 2002;**2**:465-469. DOI: 10.1038/nrc818

[58] Szabo E, Riffe ME, Steinberg SM, Birrer MJ, Linnoila RI. Altered cJUN expression: An early event in human lung carcinogenesis. Cancer Research. 1996;**56**:305-315

[59] Vleugel MM, Greijer AE, Bos R, van der Wall E, van Diest PJ. c-Jun activation is associated with proliferation and angiogenesis in invasive breast cancer. Human Pathology. 2006;**37**:668-674. DOI: 10.1016/j.humpath.2006.01.022

[60] Behrens A, Sibilia M, Wagner EF. Amino-terminal phosphorylation of c-Jun regulates stress-induced apoptosis and cellular proliferation. Nature Genetics. 1999;**21**:326-329. DOI: 10.1038/6854

[61] Matsuzaki H, Daitoku H, Hatta M, Tanaka K, Fukamizu A. Insulin-induced phosphorylation of FKHR (Foxo1) targets to proteasomal degradation. Proceedings of the National Academy of Sciences. 2003;**100**:11285-11290. DOI: 10.1073/pnas.1934283100

[62] Lu H, Huang H. FOXO1: A potential target for human diseases. Current Drug Targets [Internet]. 2011 [cited 15 Sep 2018]. Available: http://www.eurekaselect.com/74460/article

[63] Farhan M, Wang H, Gaur U, Little PJ, Xu J, Zheng W. FOXO signaling pathways as therapeutic targets in cancer. International Journal of Biological Sciences. 2017;**13**:815-827. DOI: 10.7150/ijbs.20052

[64] Fu Z, Tindall D. FOXOs, cancer and regulation of apoptosis. Oncogene. 2008;**27**:2312. DOI: 10.1038/onc.2008.24

[65] Zhang Y, Zhang L, Sun H, Lv Q, Qiu C, Che X, et al. Forkhead transcription factor 1 inhibits endometrial cancer cell proliferation via sterol regulatory element-binding protein 1. Oncology Letters. 2017;**13**:731-737. DOI: 10.3892/ol.2016.5480

[66] Zhang X, Tang N, Hadden TJ, Rishi AK. Akt, FoxO and regulation of apoptosis. Biochimica et Biophysica Acta (BBA)—Molecular Cell Research. 2011;**1813**:1978-1986. DOI: 10.1016/j.bbamcr.2011.03.010

[67] Ratnayake W, Apostolatos C, Breedy S, Apostolatos A, Acevedo-Duncan M. FOXO1 regulates oncogenic PKC-ι expression in melanoma inversely to c-Jun in an autocrine manner via IL-17E and ICAM-1 activation. World Academy of Sciences Journal. 2018;**1**(1):25-38. DOI: 10.3892/wasj.2018.2

[68] Wisdom R, Johnson RS, Moore C. c-Jun regulates cell cycle progression and apoptosis by distinct mechanisms. The EMBO Journal. 1999;**18**:188-197. DOI: 10.1093/emboj/18.1.188

[69] Hodge DR, Hurt EM, Farrar WL. The role of IL-6 and STAT3 in inflammation and cancer. European Journal of Cancer. 2005;**41**:2502-2512. DOI: 10.1016/j.ejca.2005.08.016

[70] Yue P, Turkson J. Targeting STAT3 in cancer: How successful are we? Expert Opinion on Investigational Drugs. 2009;**18**:45-56. DOI: 10.1517/13543780802565791

[71] Page BDG, Khoury H, Laister RC, Fletcher S, Vellozo M, Manzoli A, et al. Small molecule STAT5-SH2 domain inhibitors exhibit potent antileukemia activity. Journal of Medicinal Chemistry. 2012;**55**:1047-1055. DOI: 10.1021/jm200720n

[72] Pardanani A, Lasho T, Smith G, Burns CJ, Fantino E, Tefferi A. CYT387, a selective JAK1/JAK2 inhibitor: *In vitro* assessment of kinase selectivity and preclinical studies using cell lines and primary cells from polycythemia vera patients. Leukemia. 2009;**23**:1441-1445. DOI: 10.1038/leu.2009.50

[73] Korneev KV, Atretkhany K-SN, Drutskaya MS, Grivennikov SI,

Kuprash DV, Nedospasov SA. TLR-signaling and proinflammatory cytokines as drivers of tumorigenesis. Cytokine. 2017;**89**:127-135. DOI: 10.1016/j.cyto.2016.01.021

[74] Zhang X, Wrzeszczynska MH, Horvath CM, Darnell JE. Interacting regions in Stat3 and c-Jun that participate in cooperative transcriptional activation. Molecular and Cellular Biology. 1999;**19**:7138-7146

[75] Hornsveld M, Dansen TB, Derksen PW, Burgering BMT. Re-evaluating the role of FOXOs in cancer. Seminars in Cancer Biology. 2018;**50**:90-100. DOI: 10.1016/j.semcancer.2017.11.017

[76] Sunters A, Madureira PA, Pomeranz KM, Aubert M, Brosens JJ, Cook SJ, et al. Paclitaxel-induced nuclear translocation of FOXO3a in breast cancer cells is mediated by c-Jun NH2-terminal kinase and Akt. Cancer Research. 2006;**66**:212-220. DOI: 10.1158/0008-5472.CAN-05-1997

[77] Antonicelli F, Lorin J, Kurdykowski S, Gangloff SC, Naour RL, Sallenave JM, et al. CXCL10 reduces melanoma proliferation and invasiveness in vitro and in vivo. The British Journal of Dermatology. 2011;**164**:720-728. DOI: 10.1111/j.1365-2133.2010.10176.x

[78] Zaynagetdinov R, Sherrill TP, Gleaves LA, McLoed AG, Saxon JA, Habermann AC, et al. Interleukin-5 facilitates lung metastasis by modulating the immune microenvironment. Cancer Research. 2015;**75**:1624-1634. DOI: 10.1158/0008-5472.CAN-14-2379

[79] Ishiguro H, Akimoto K, Nagashima Y, Kojima Y, Sasaki T, Ishiguro-Imagawa Y, et al. aPKCλ/ι promotes growth of prostate cancer cells in an autocrine manner through transcriptional activation of interleukin-6. Proceedings of the National Academy of Sciences. 2009;**106**:16369-16374. DOI: 10.1073/pnas.0907044106

[80] Peng H, Chen P, Cai Y, Chen Y, Wu Q, Li Y, et al. Endothelin-1 increases expression of cyclooxygenase-2 and production of interlukin-8 in Hunan pulmonary epithelial cells. Peptides. 2008;**29**:419-424. DOI: 10.1016/j.peptides.2007.11.015

[81] Timani KA, Győrffy B, Liu Y, Mohammad KS, He JJ. Tip110/SART3 regulates IL-8 expression and predicts the clinical outcomes in melanoma. Molecular Cancer. 2018;**17**:1-6. DOI: 10.1186/s12943-018-0868-z

[82] Yang M, Liu J, Piao C, Shao J, Du J. ICAM-1 suppresses tumor metastasis by inhibiting macrophage M2 polarization through blockade of efferocytosis. Cell Death & Disease. 2015;**6**:e1780. DOI: 10.1038/cddis.2015.144

[83] de Groote ML, Kazemier HG, Huisman C, van der Gun BTF, Faas MM, Rots MG. Upregulation of endogenous ICAM-1 reduces ovarian cancer cell growth in the absence of immune cells. International Journal of Cancer. 2014;**134**:280-290. DOI: 10.1002/ijc.28375

[84] Benatar T, Cao MY, Lee Y, Lightfoot J, Feng N, Gu X, et al. IL-17E, a proinflammatory cytokine, has antitumor efficacy against several tumor types in vivo. Cancer Immunology, Immunotherapy. 2010;**59**:805-817. DOI: 10.1007/s00262-009-0802-8

[85] Benatar T, Cao MY, Lee Y, Li H, Feng N, Gu X, et al. Virulizin induces production of IL-17E to enhance antitumor activity by recruitment of eosinophils into tumors. Cancer Immunology, Immunotherapy. 2008;**57**:1757-1769. DOI: 10.1007/s00262-008-0502-9

[86] Wei C, Sirikanjanapong S, Lieberman S, Delacure M, Martiniuk F, Levis W, et al. Primary mucosal melanoma arising from the eustachian

tube with CTLA-4, IL-17A, IL-17C, and IL-17E upregulation. Ear, Nose, & Throat Journal. 2013;**92**:36-40

[87] Stallings-Mann M, Jamieson L, Regala RP, Weems C, Murray NR, Fields AP. A novel small-molecule inhibitor of protein kinase Cι blocks transformed growth of non–small-cell lung cancer cells. Cancer Research. 2006;**66**: 1767-1774. DOI: 10.1158/0008-5472. CAN-05-3405

[88] Blázquez AB, Vázquez-Calvo Á, Martín-Acebes MA, Saiz J-C. Pharmacological inhibition of protein kinase C reduces West Nile virus replication. Viruses. 2018;**10**:91. DOI: 10.3390/v10020091

[89] Kim HK, Cho SW, Heo HJ, Jeong SH, Kim M, Ko KS, et al. A novel atypical PKC-iota inhibitor, Echinochrome a, enhances Cardiomyocyte differentiation from mouse embryonic stem cells. Marine Drugs. 2018;**16**:192. DOI: 10.3390/md16060192

[90] Kwiatkowski J, Liu B, Tee DHY, Chen G, Ahmad NHB, Wong YX, et al. Fragment-based drug discovery of potent protein kinase C iota inhibitors. Journal of Medicinal Chemistry. 2018;**61**:4386-4396. DOI: 10.1021/acs. jmedchem.8b00060

Chapter 3

Hormonal Regulation of Cutaneous Melanoma: A Brief Review of In Vivo and In Vitro Studies and Its Clinical Implication

Pandurangan Ramaraj

Abstract

Skin is an endocrine organ. Skin produces various hypothalamic, pituitary, adrenal and sex steroid hormones. This raises the question whether skin cancer melanoma is a hormone dependent cancer. But, a review of in-vivo and in-vitro studies suggested that melanoma could be a hormone responsive cancer or hormone sensitive cancer. In fact, previous clinical study showed that menstruating females were better protected in melanoma than post-menopausal women and men of any age. However, the study did not show any direct effect of steroid hormone on melanoma cells. Our in-vitro study showed that progesterone, a female sex hormone significantly inhibited human melanoma (BLM) cell growth. Progesterone inhibitory effect on other melanoma cell lines was also reported by Fang et al., Moroni et al. and Kanda and Watanbe. So, it was hypothesized that progesterone could be protecting menstruating females in melanoma. Our further research showed that progesterone action was mediated by a specific suppression of pro-inflammatory cytokine IL-8. Several in-vivo and in-vitro studies showed the importance of IL-8 in the regulation of melanoma growth. Hence, IL-8 could be considered as a potential target for melanoma treatment.

Keywords: skin, steroid hormones, melanoma, in vivo and in vitro studies, progesterone, IL-8

1. Introduction

The skin is not only a target organ for sex hormones [1] but also an endocrine organ. The skin produces sex hormones, viz., androgens, estrogen, and progestins, which function locally [2, 3]. Weak androgens such as dehydroepiandrosterone (DHEA), DHEA sulfate (DHEAS), and androstenedione are converted to more potent testosterone and 5-α-dihydrotestosterone in the skin [4]. In addition, the skin has all the elements of neuroendocrine axis with the expression of corticotrophin-releasing hormone (CRH), pro-opiomelanocortin (POMC), and associated peptides ACTH, α-melanocyte-stimulating hormone (MSH), β-endorphin, and corticotrophin-releasing hormone receptor-1 [5, 6]. The presence of receptor and the peptides in the same cell suggests auto-, para-, and intracrine functions of these axes. The skin has nervous and hormonal pathways not only to regulate itself but also to regulate systemic homeostasis. Imbalances in hormones affect skin texture and cause skin diseases such as rosacea, atopic dermatitis, and psoriasis [7, 8]. Melanoma is one such fatal disorder or disease of the skin [9], which is believed to be caused by UV rays [10]. According to the Cancer Society Report, melanoma is on the rise. In 2018 alone 91,720 new cases would be diagnosed in the United States with an estimated 9000 deaths in the United States alone [11]. It has been shown that sex steroids are essential for a healthy skin. Since melanoma is a serious skin disease, the question, whether melanoma is a hormone dependent cancer or not is relevant here. Literature survey showed possible dependence of melanoma on endocrine influences [12–14]. Several in vivo and in vitro studies showed the involvement of steroids in the regulation of melanoma growth.

2. Brief review of in vivo studies

2.1 Animal studies

Animal studies showed the involvement of sex steroid hormones in the regulation of melanoma growth, and there were also differences in the regulation of growth between male and female mice:

a. In one study, estrogen receptor-positive human melanoma cells grew more slowly in female than in male mice [15].

b. Female survival benefit with metastatic melanoma was observed, when melanoma cells produced liver metastases preferentially in male compared to female mice [16].

c. In another study, dihydrotestosterone was shown to stimulate proliferation, whereas anti-androgen receptor hydroxyflutamide [17] showed anticancer action in a male mouse transplanted with melanoma.

In the following two studies, it was shown that male mice were more prone to cancer than female mice:

d. When induced with carcinogen [18].

e. When exposed to UV-B [19].

2.2 Clinical studies

Overall survival outcome for young women (45 years of age and under) was far superior to older women (55 years of age and older) and men of any age group [20]. A 22% survival advantage and 17% 5 year disease-free interval advantage were observed in females [21]. In addition, women were found to survive longer than men after the development of stage III disease [22]. Clinical studies also suggested the involvement of hormones in the regulation of melanoma growth. So, clinical studies underlined the involvement of female sex steroid hormones in protecting menstruating females in melanoma. But, these clinical studies did not identify the exact female hormone involved in the protection. In addition, there was no statistically significant difference observed in the survival rates between controls and women diagnosed with melanoma stage I or stage II during pregnancy [23–25]. Data also showed no correlation between melanoma and oral contraceptives

[26, 27]. Available data suggested no connection between exogenous hormones and the risk for malignant melanoma [28, 29].

3. Brief review of in vitro studies

The following in vitro studies showed inhibitory effect of steroid hormones on a variety of melanoma cell lines, suggesting melanoma could be a hormone-sensitive cancer:

a. 2-Methoxyestradiol (2-ME), an estrogenic metabolite, inhibited all tested melanoma cell line growth, without affecting the growth of non-tumorigenic cells [30].

b. Kanda and Watanbe showed that 17-β-estradiol, progesterone, and dihydrotestosterone inhibited melanoma cell growth in a receptor-dependent manner by suppressing IL-8 transcription [31].

c. Amelanotic strain cells grew faster in vivo in female hamsters [32], whereas testosterone inhibited the cell growth in vitro.

d. Glucocorticoids also showed their effect on melanoma cell growth in a receptor-dependent manner [33].

e. Another in vitro study showed that melatonin at physiological concentrations (1 nM to 10 pM) inhibited metastatic mouse melanoma (B16BL6) cell growth [34].

4. In vitro studies from our lab

Our lab in vitro studies showed involvement of progesterone in the regulation of mouse and human melanoma cell growth.

4.1 Dose-response studies of progesterone with mouse (B16F10) and human melanoma (BLM) cell line

Initially four sex steroids, viz., dehydroepiandrosterone (DHEA), androstenedione (AD), testosterone (T), and progesterone (P4), were checked for their effect on mouse melanoma (B16F10) cell growth [35]. Though all four steroids showed a dose-dependent effect, progesterone showed a significant effect on the inhibition of mouse melanoma cell growth (**Figure 1**). As the initial study was carried out at high concentrations (100, 150, and 200 μM), dose-response study was carried out to rule out toxic effect of high concentrations of steroids on melanoma cell growth inhibition. Mouse (B16F10) and human melanoma (BLM) cells showed a dose-dependent cell growth inhibition [35, 36], suggesting the inhibition was not due to toxic effect at high concentration of steroids (**Figure 1**).

4.2 Mechanism of inhibition of human melanoma (BLM) cell growth

After having ruled out necrosis and apoptosis as the cause of cell growth inhibition, it was found out that autophagy was the mechanism of cell growth inhibition (**Figure 2**), using a known inducer of autophagy (spermidine) in a control experiment [36].

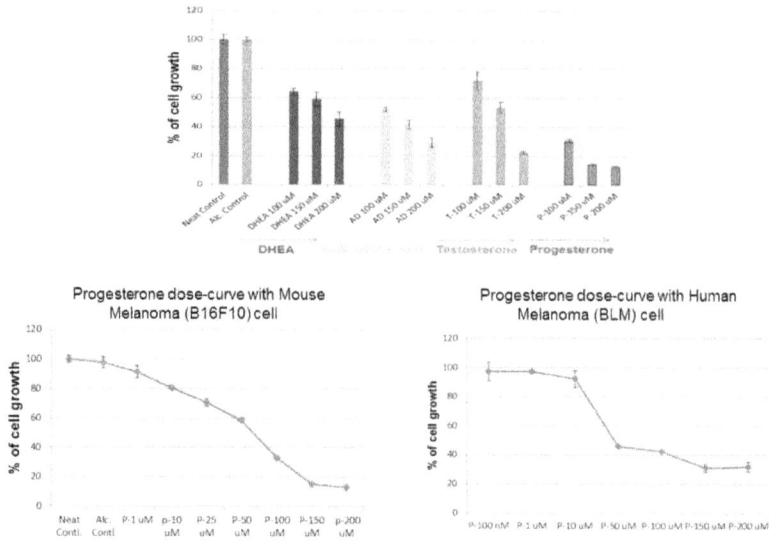

Figure 1.

Dose-response studies of progesterone with mouse (B16F10) and human melanoma (BLM) cell lines. Initially dehydroepiandrosterone, androstenedione, testosterone, and progesterone were tested for their effects on mouse melanoma (B16F10) cell growth by MTT assay. Progesterone, a female sex hormone, showed significant inhibition at 150 and 200 μM concentrations. As steroids were tested initially at high concentrations (100, 150, and 200 μM), dose-response study was carried out to rule out toxic effect of steroid at high concentrations. Dose-response studies of mouse (B16F10) and human melanoma (BLM) cell lines showed a sigmoidal dose-response curve, ruling out toxic effect of steroids due to high concentrations.

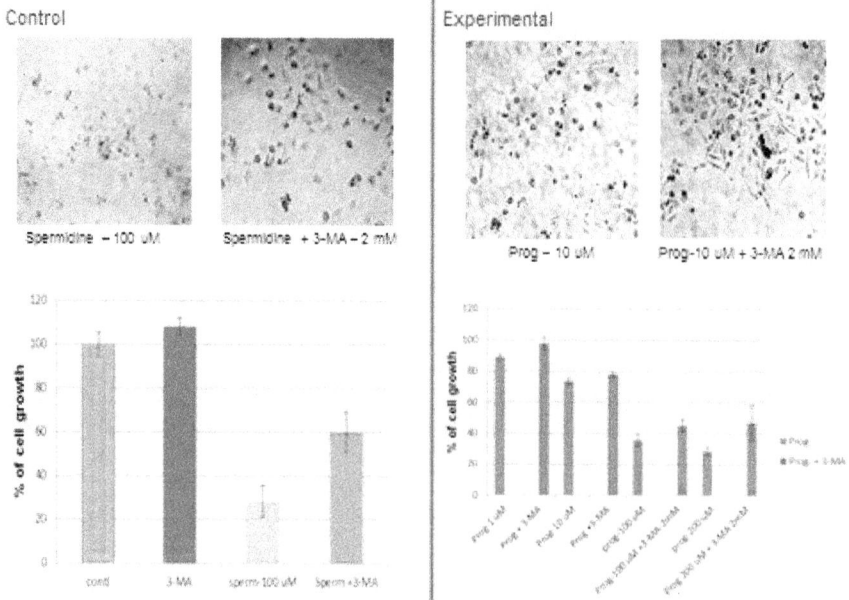

Figure 2.

Mechanism of cell death by progesterone. After having ruled out necrosis and apoptosis, autophagy was checked by adding 3-methyladenine (3-MA). Control experiment with 100 μM of spermidine-induced autophagy was partially rescued by the addition of 2 mM of 3-methyladenine (as 3-MA inhibited the assembly of autophagosome formation [37, 38]). Similar partial rescue of cell growth was observed at various concentrations of progesterone, suggesting the mechanism of inhibition of cell growth was due to autophagy.

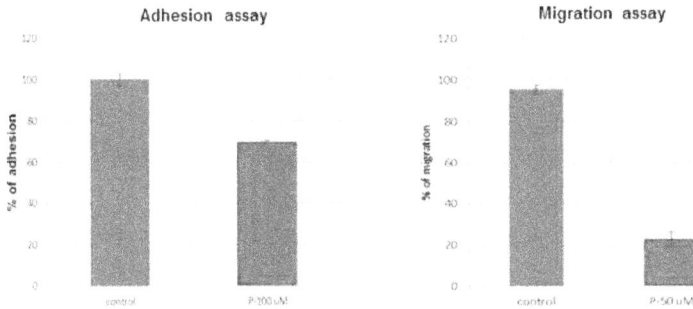

Figure 3.
In vitro adhesion and migration functions of human melanoma cell line. Human melanoma cells were treated with progesterone at 100 μM for 48 h in petri dish. After 48 h, both control and progesterone-treated cells were harvested, and adhesion assay was carried out as per the protocol in Ref. [28]. For migration assay, control and progesterone (50 μM)-treated cells were harvested after 48 h of treatment. Adhesion experiment showed partial inhibition of adhesion in progesterone-treated cells compared to untreated control cells. Similarly, progesterone-treated cells showed a significant decrease in migration function in progesterone-treated cells compared to untreated control cells.

4.3 Effect of progesterone on adhesion and migration functions of human melanoma cells

Effects on adhesion and migration functions were checked after 48 h incubation of human melanoma cells with progesterone. Progesterone at 100 μM concentration partially inhibited adhesion function (**Figure 3**). Similarly, progesterone (50 μM) treatment significantly decreased migration function of human melanoma cells (**Figure 3**). This study indicated that progesterone treatment decreased adhesion and migration functions [39] which were essential for metastasis of melanoma.

5. In vitro studies from other labs

In addition, in vitro inhibition of melanoma cell growth by progesterone was also shown by other labs:

a. Fang et al. showed inhibition of human melanoma cell lines (A375, A875) by progesterone and RU-486, which were not mediated through progesterone receptor [40].

b. Moroni et al. repeated the studies with A375 cell line and used progesterone concentration up to 1000 μM, which also showed inhibition of human melanoma cell growth [41].

c. Kanda and Watanbe used progesterone along with dihydrotestosterone and estrogen and showed that all the three steroids inhibited human melanoma cell growth by decreasing IL-8 transcription [31].

6. Biochemical basis of progesterone action

Further research [42] involving ELISArray of supernatants of the cells treated with progesterone along with untreated control cells showed that progesterone action was mediated by a specific suppression pro-inflammatory cytokine IL8 (**Figure 4**).

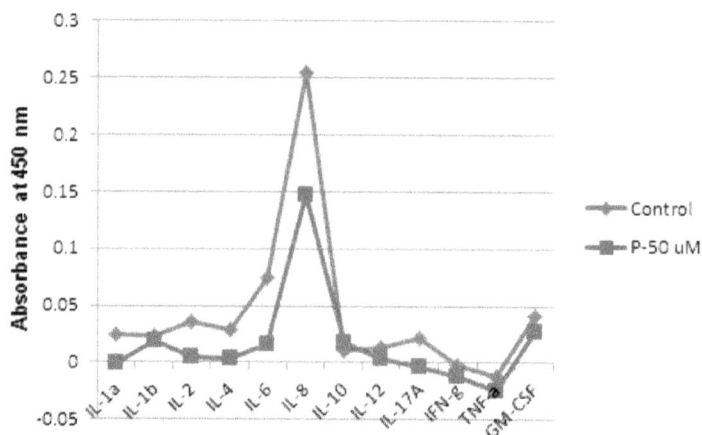

Figure 4.
Biochemical basis of progesterone action. An ELISArray, containing pro- and anti-inflammatory cytokine antibodies coated in different wells, showed a specific suppression of IL-8 cytokine alone in the supernatant of cells treated with progesterone (50 µM) compared to untreated control cell supernatant.

6.1 Involvement of IL-8 in melanoma growth

In vivo and in vitro studies from other labs showed the involvement of IL-8 in melanoma growth:

1. IL-8 cytokine produced in vitro was an essential autocrine growth factor for melanoma cells [43].

2. Expression of IL-8 in human melanoma cells upregulated the activity of matrix metalloproteinase (MMP) and increased tumor growth and metastasis [44].

3. Expression of IL-8 correlated with metastatic potential of human melanoma cell in nude mouse [45].

7. Summary

In vivo and in vitro studies showed the inhibition of melanoma growth by various hormones. This inhibition of cell growth by various hormones suggested that melanoma could be a hormone-responsive cancer, where hormones were essential for survival in melanoma. This was supported by the clinical studies carried out in the 1950s and 1960s. One clinical study reported that menstruating females were better protected in melanoma than postmenopausal women and men of any age [20]. But, the study did not correlate with steroid status of females. Literature showed that progesterone level peaked in menstruating females between 1000 and 1500 ng/dl, whereas progesterone level ranged between 20 and 100 ng/dl in postmenopausal women [46]. Our research also showed that progesterone inhibited human melanoma (BLM) cell growth in vitro significantly. In addition, progesterone inhibitory action was also shown by Fang et al., Moroni et al., and Kanda and Watanbe. So, it was hypothesized that progesterone could be protecting menstruating females. Recently, it was shown that the protective function of progesterone was mediated by a specific suppression of pro-inflammatory cytokine IL-8. Various in vitro and in vivo studies already showed the importance of IL-8 in melanoma cell growth.

8. Conclusion

Several studies showed the involvement of progesterone in the regulation of in vitro melanoma cell growth and also in the regulation of in vivo melanoma growth. Further in vitro research showed that the progesterone inhibitory action was mediated by a specific suppression of pro-inflammatory cytokine IL-8. The connection between IL-8 and melanoma growth was already established by other investigators. This brought IL-8 into focus in melanoma and suggested that IL-8 could be considered as a potential target for melanoma treatment.

Author details

Pandurangan Ramaraj
Department of Biochemistry, Kirksville College of Osteopathic Medicine, A.T. Still University of Health Sciences, Kirksville, MO, USA

*Address all correspondence to: pramaraj@atsu.edu

IntechOpen

References

[1] Zouboulis CC. The human skin as a hormone target and an endocrine gland. Hormones. 2004;**3**(1):9-26

[2] Zouboulis CC. Human skin: An independent peripheral endocrine organ. Hormone Research. 2000;**54**:230-242

[3] Zouboulis CC, Chen WC, Thornton MJ, Qin K, Rosenfield R. Sexual hormones in human skin. Hormone and Metabolic Research. 2007;**39**(2):85-95

[4] Labrie F. DHEA and its transformation into androgens and estrogens in peripheral target tissues: Intracrinology. Frontiers in Neuroendocrinology. 2001;**22**(3):185-212

[5] Slominski A, Wortsman J. Neuroendocrinology of the skin. Endocrine Reviews. 2000;**21**(5):457-487

[6] Slominski A, Wortsman J. Self-regulated endocrine systems in the skin. Minerva Endocrinologica. 2003;**28**(2):135-143

[7] Slominski A, Zbytek B, Nikolakis G, Manna PR, Skobowiat C, Zmijewski M, et al. Steroidogenesis in the skin: Implications for local immune functions. The Journal of Steroid Biochemistry and Molecular Biology. 2013;**137**:107-123. DOI: 10.1016/j.jsbmb.2013.02.006. Epub 2013 Feb19

[8] Nikolakis G, Stratakis CA, Kanaki T, Slominski A, Zouboulis CC. Skin steroidogenesis in health and disease. Reviews in Endocrine & Metabolic Disorders. 2016;**17**(3):247-258

[9] Gray-Schopfer V, Wellbrock C, Marais R. Melanoma biology and new targeted therapy. Nature. 2007;**445**:851-857

[10] Rass K, Reicharth J. UV damage and DNA repair in malignant melanoma and non-melanoma skin cancer.

Advances in Experimental Medicine and Biology. 2008;**624**:162-178. DOI: 10.1007/978-0-387-77574-6_13

[11] Available from: http://seer.cancer.gov/statfacts/html/melan.html

[12] Sadoff L, Winkley J, Tyson S. Is malignant melanoma an endocrine-dependent tumor? Oncology. 1973;**27**:244-257

[13] Gupta A, Driscoll MS. Do hormones influence melanoma? Facts and controversies. Clinics in Dermatology. 2010;**28**(3):287-292

[14] De Giorgi V, Gori A, Alfaioli B, Papi F, Grazzini M, Rossari S, et al. Influence of sex hormones on melanoma. Journal of Clinical Oncology. 2011;**29**(4):e94-e95

[15] Feucht KA, Walker MJ, Das Gupta TK, Beattie CW. Effect of 17-β-oestradiol on the growth of estrogen receptor positive human melanoma in vitro and in athymic mice. Cancer Research. 1988;**48**:7093-7101

[16] Ladanyi A, Timar J, Bocsi J, Towari J, Lapis K. Sex-dependent liver metastasis of human melanoma lines in SCID mice. Melanoma Research. 1995;**5**:83-86

[17] Morvillo V, Luthy IA, Bravo AI, Capurro MI, Donaldson M, Quintans C, et al. Atypical androgen receptor in the human melanoma cell line IIB-MEL-J. Pigment Cell Research. 1995;**8**(3):135-141

[18] Simanainen U, Ryan T, Li D, Suarez FG, Gao YR, Watson G, et al. Androgen receptor actions modify skin structure and chemical carcinogen-induced skin cancer susceptibility in mice. Hormones and Cancer. 2015;**6**:45-53

[19] Thomas-Ahner JM, Wulff BC, Tober KL, Kusewitt DF, Riggenbach JA,

Oberyszyn TM. Gender differences in UV-B induced skin carcinogenesis, inflammation and DNA damage. Cancer Research. 2007;**67**(7): 3468-3474. DOI: 10.1158/0008-5472. CAN-06-3798

[20] Kemeny MM, Busch E, Stewart AK, Mench HR. Superior survival of young women with malignant melanoma. American Journal of Surgery. 1988;**175**:437-444

[21] Miller JG, Neil SM. Gender and cutaneous melanoma. The British Journal of Dermatology. 1997;**136**:657-665

[22] Rumke P, Kleeberg UR, Mackie RM, Lejeune FJ, Planting AS, Brocker EB, et al. Tamoxifen as a single agent for advanced melanoma in postmenopausal women. A phase II study of the EORTC malignant melanoma cooperative group. Melanoma Research. 1992;**2**:153-156

[23] Smith MA, Fine JA, Barnhill RL, Berwick M. Hormonal and reproductive influences and risk of melanoma in women. International Journal of Epidemiology. 1998;**27**(5):751-757

[24] Miller E, Barnea Y, Gur E, Leshem D, Karin E, Weiss J, et al. Malignant melanoma and pregnancy: Second thoughts. Journal of Plastic, Reconstructive & Aesthetic Surgery. 2010;**63**(7):1163-1168. DOI: 10.1016/j. bjps.2009.05.050

[25] Schaepkens van Riempst J, Abdou M, Schertenleib P. Melanoma: A protective role of pregnancy? A case report and review of literature. (Article in French). Annales de Chirurgie Plastique et Esthétique. 2011;**56**(1):43-48

[26] Leslie KK, Espey E. Oral contraceptives and skin cancer: Is there a link? American Journal of Clinical Dermatology. 2005;**6**(6):349-355

[27] Hannaford PC, Villard-Mackintosh L, Vessey MP, Kay CR. Oral contraceptives and malignant melanoma. British Journal of Cancer. 1991;**63**(3):430-433

[28] Durvasula R, Ahmed SM, Vashisht A, Studd JW. Hormone replacement therapy and malignant melanoma: To prescribe or not to prescribe? Climacteric. 2002;**5**(2):197-200

[29] Tang JY, Spaunhurst KM, Chlebowski RT, Wactawski-Wende J, Fridtjof Thomas EK, Anderson ML, et al. Menopausal hormone therapy and risks of melanoma and nonmelanoma skin cancers: Women's health initiative randaomized trials. Journal of the National Cancer Institute. 2011;**103**(19):1469-1475

[30] Ghosh R, Ott AM, Seetharam D, Slaga TJ, Kumar AP. Cell cycle block and apoptosis induction in a human melanoma cell line following treatment with 2-methoxyostradiol: Therapeutic implications? Melanoma Research. 2003;**13**(2):119-127

[31] Kanda N, Watanbe S. 17-β-estradiol, progesterone and dihydrotestosterone suppress the growth of human melanoma by inhibiting interleukin-8 production. The Journal of Investigative Dermatology. 2001;**117**:274-283

[32] Lipkin G. Sex factors in growth of malignant melanoma in hamsters: In vivo and in vitro correlation. Cancer Research. 1970;**30**:1928-1930

[33] Disorbo DM, McNulty B, Nathanson L. In vitro growth inhibition of human malignant melanoma cells by glucocorticoids. Cancer Research. 1983;**43**:2664-2667

[34] Cos S, Garcia-Bolado A, Sanchez-Barcelo E. Direct antiproliferative effects of melatonin on two metastatic

cell sub-lines of mouse melanoma (B16BL6 and PG19). Melanoma Research. 2001;**11**(2):197-201

[35] Ramaraj P, Cox JL. In vitro effect of sex steroids on mouse melanoma (B16F10) cell growth. CellBio. 2014;**3**: 60-71. DOI: 10.4236/cellbio.2014.32007

[36] Ramaraj P, Cox JL. In vitro effect of progesterone on human melanoma (BLM) cell growth. International Journal of Clinical and Experimental Medicine. 2014;7(11):3941-3953, PMID: 25550902; PMCID: PMC4276160

[37] Seglen PO, Gordon PB. 3-Methyladenine: Specific inhibitor of autophagic/lysosomal protein degradation in isolated rat hepatocytes. Proceedings of the National Academy of Sciences of the United States of America. 1982;**79**:1889-1892

[38] Jagannath C, Lindsey DR, Dhandayuthapani S, Xu Y, Hunter RL Jr, Eissa NT. Autophagy enhances the efficacy of BCG vaccine by increasing peptide presentation in mouse dendritic cells. Nature Medicine. 2009;**15**(3):267-276

[39] Leder DC, Brown JR, Ramaraj P. In vitro rescue and recovery studies of human melanoma (BLM) cell growth, adhesion and migration functions after treatment with progesterone. International Journal of Clinical and Experimental Medicine. 2015;**8**(8):12275-12285. PMID: 26550137 [PubMed] PMCID: PMC4612822

[40] Fang X, Zhang X, Zhou M, Li J. Effects of progesterone on the growth regulation in classical progesterone receptor-negative malignant melanoma cells. Journal of Huazhong University of Science and Technology. Medical Sciences. 2010;**30**(2):231-234. DOI: 10.1007/s 11596-010-0220-3

[41] Moroni G, Gaziano R, Bue C, Agostini M, Perno CF,

Sinibaldi-Vallebona P, et al. Progesterone and melanoma cells: An old story suspended between life and death. Journal of Steroids and Hormonal Science. 2015;**S13**:158. DOI: 10.4172/2157-7536.1000158

[42] Miller A, Fulcher A, Dock P, Ramaraj P. Biochemical basis of protection by progesterone in melanoma based on curcumin pre-treatment of human melanoma cell models. In: Endo2018Home; 2018. Available from: http://www.abstractsonline.com/ pp8/#!/4482/presentation/7469

[43] Schadendorf D, Möller A, Algermissen B, Worm M, Sticherling M, Czarnetzki BM. IL-8 produced by human malignant melanoma cells in vitro is an essential autocrine growth factor. Journal of Immunology. 1993;**151**(5):2667-2675

[44] Luca M, Huang S, Gershenwald JE, Singh RK, Reich R, Bar-Eli M. Expression of interleukin-8 by human melanoma cells up-regulates MMP-2 activity and increases tumor growth and metastasis. The American Journal of Pathology. 1997;**151**(4):1105-1113

[45] Singh RK, Gutman M, Radinsky R, Bucana CD, Fidler IJ. Expression of interleukin 8 correlates with the metastatic potential of human melanoma cells in nude mice. Cancer Research. 1994;**54**(12):3242-3247

[46] Häggström M. Reference ranges for estradiol, progesterone, luteinizing hormone and follicle-stimulating hormone during the menstrual cycle. WikiJournal of Medicine. 2014;**1**(1):1. DOI: 10.15347/wjm/2014.001

Section 2

Special Melanoma Scenarios

Chapter 4

Melanoma and Pregnancy: Risks, Current, and Forecast

Ignatko Irina Vladimirovna and

Strizhakov Alexander Nikolaevich

Abstract

Currently, the term "melanoma associated with pregnancy" is used, implying the inclusion of all clinical observations of melanoma diagnosis during pregnancy and in the first 2 years after delivery. The management of pregnant women with newly diagnosed melanoma is likewise controversial, especially with regard to the management of women with an advanced melanoma. Thrombotic complications are the most common form of paraneoplastic syndrome, which largely determines the prognosis of the disease. The presented chapter is intended to familiarize practical physicians with the complexities that arise in the management of pregnant women with a developing metastatic disease, with questions of the progression of the disease during pregnancy, with the emergence of severe paraneoplastic complications involving secondary thrombophilia, amaranthine endocarditis, and widespread arterial thrombosis. The possibility of using modern antitumor drugs (Zelboraf) is shown. It is emphasized that in the management of such patients, the need for an effective team of specialists of various profiles is especially high: oncologists, obstetrician-gynecologists, surgeons, hematologists, anesthesiologist-resuscitators, and US and magnetic resonance imaging (MRI) diagnostics.

Keywords: melanoma, pregnancy, secondary thrombophilia, paraneoplastic syndrome, vemurafenib

1. Introduction

Melanoma of the skin (*lat. —melanoma, melanoma malignum*) is a malignant tumor that results from neoplastic transformation of melanocytes—cells that produce various variations of melanin pigment [1]. In recent years, there has been an increase in the incidence of skin melanoma in Russia. Between 1998 and 2008, the incidence rate in the Russian Federation was 38.17%, and the standardized morbidity rate rose from 4.04 to 5.46 per 100,000 population. In 2008, the number of new cases of melanoma in the Russian Federation was 7744 people. Mortality from melanoma in the Russian Federation in 2008 was 3159 people and a standardized death rate of 2.23 people per 100,000 population [2]. Approximately one-third of women diagnosed with melanoma are of childbearing age, and a 2015 Swedish population-based cancer registry study found that melanoma was the most common malignancy in pregnancy [3]. Melanoma is a significant proportion of all tumors diagnosed during pregnancy, and this figure is up to 25% among all tumor diseases during gestation. There is continuing controversy concerning the prognosis of women diagnosed with melanoma during pregnancy. Initial concerns about pregnancy's impact on prognosis in women diagnosed with melanoma date back to case reports from the 1950s. These reports suggested that pregnancy might lead to transformation of nevi into melanomas, increase the growth rate of existing melanomas, and cause localized melanomas to metastasize [4]. Subsequently, multiple observations seemed to support the argument that melanoma is a hormonally responsive malignancy: changes in skin pigmentation during pregnancy, detection of hormone receptors on some melanomas using older technology, a higher incidence of melanoma after puberty, and relative immunosuppression during pregnancy. The management of women diagnosed with melanoma during pregnancy is likewise controversial, particularly concerning sentinel lymph node biopsy (SLNB) and decisions about the management of the patient with nodal or metastatic disease [5]. Multiple studies have looked at the relationship between pregnancy and cutaneous melanoma. Factors limiting the interpretation of the literature include the following:

- Many of the case series prior to the 1980s did not account for the most important prognostic factors, such as depth of tumor or stage of disease. Subsequently, there have been a number of small case-control studies and large population-based cohort studies. While the case-control studies have the advantage of including important prognostic factors, the small numbers of patients included are an important limitation. Conversely, the larger cohort studies lack complete data on staging and Breslow depth.

- Some of the larger studies do not distinguish between diagnosis of melanoma during pregnancy and diagnosis during the postpartum period. Such studies refer to these patients as having pregnancy-associated melanoma (PAM). The definition of PAM varies in different studies and ranges from diagnosis during pregnancy to diagnosis up to 5 years after delivery [6].

- There is significant variability in the techniques and quality of the statistical analysis of the data between studies and in the presence of age-matched nonpregnant control groups, as well as a lack of consideration of important confounding factors, including but not limited to age, anatomic site of lesion, sun exposure or season at time of diagnosis, depth of the melanoma, the absence or presence of ulceration, and the presence as well as number of mitoses per mm^2 [2].

2. Definition

Deciding on the role of pregnancy in the development of melanoma is important, as more women are planning a pregnancy from 30 to 40 years, and an increase in the number of melanoma diagnoses during fetal growth is expected [3, 4]. Currently, the term "melanoma associated with pregnancy" is used, implying the inclusion of all clinical observations of the diagnosis of melanoma during pregnancy and in the first 2 years after delivery [5].

2.1 Diagnosis prior to pregnancy

Few studies have addressed the impact on prognosis when melanoma is diagnosed before a woman becomes pregnant, but based upon the available data, there does not appear to be an effect on prognosis. In a large Swedish retrospective cohort study [6], 966 women who had pregnancies after a diagnosis of a primary melanoma were compared with 4567 women who did not become pregnant after diagnosis. After adjustment for Breslow depth, tumor site, Clark level, and age, pregnancy did not significantly affect survival (HR 0.58, 95% CI 0.32–1.05). For patients with a history of melanoma and multiple dysplastic nevi, we suggest more frequent dermatology examinations during pregnancy [7].

2.2 Diagnosis during pregnancy

Most of the multiple small controlled studies and large population-based cohort studies [6] do not show a negative influence of pregnancy on survival [2]. In a review of 10 case-control studies that included 185 women diagnosed with melanoma during pregnancy and 5348 women of the same childbearing age who were diagnosed with melanoma but were not pregnant, pregnancy did not have an impact on survival and did not increase the risk of a second melanoma [8]. The higher the parity and the younger the age of the mother at her first delivery, the lower the risk of melanoma. Thus, the authors concluded that there was no reason for physicians to recommend deferral of subsequent pregnancies in women who have been diagnosed with a stage I melanoma during a previous pregnancy [1]. A controversial study is a single-institution study that compared 41 women diagnosed with PAM with a control group of women of childbearing age who were not pregnant within 1 year of diagnosis [9]. PAM was defined as melanoma diagnosis either during pregnancy or within 1 year after delivery. After adjustment for stage, age, and location, the PAM group showed a five-, seven-, and ninefold increase in mortality, metastasis, and recurrence, respectively, when compared with controls.

2.3 Diagnosis postpartum

Multiple large population-based cohort studies [3, 10] and one small controlled study have generally found no influence on prognosis when melanoma is diagnosed up to 5 years following delivery, except for one study that observed an enhanced risk of death from melanoma in the first year postpartum, which may be due to delayed diagnosis during pregnancy. A large retrospective English study that linked data from a national cancer registry and hospital discharge data evaluated patients diagnosed with melanoma up to 5 years postpartum [10]. There was a significant increased death rate in the first year after delivery (HR 1.92, 95% CI 1.32–2.79) but not in the four subsequent years postpartum. Another study found a lower incidence of melanoma diagnosed during pregnancy than expected compared with the first 6 months postpartum [2]. The spike in melanoma diagnosis and death in the early postpartum period may be caused by a delay in diagnosis.

3. Classification

The eighth edition of the American Joint Committee on Cancer (AJCC) tumor, node, and metastasis (TNM) staging system is based upon an evaluation of the primary tumor, the regional lymph nodes and lymphatic drainage, and the presence or absence of distant metastases. The information from TNM staging is then combined to classify patients into AJCC prognostic stage groups. There are four major growth patterns of melanoma: lentigo maligna, nodular, superficial spreading, and acral lentiginous. In an observational study of close to 120,000 patients with melanoma, nodular melanoma was an independent risk factor for death, after controlling for thickness, ulceration, and stage [11]. Nevertheless, the eighth edition of the American Joint Committee on Cancer tumor, node, and metastasis staging system, which relies upon the primary tumor thickness and other features, involvement of regional lymph nodes, and presence or absence of distant metastases, should be used to stage melanomas of any growth pattern. Most melanomas arise as superficial tumors that are confined to the epidermis, where they may remain for several to many years. During this stage, known as the horizontal or "radial" growth phase, the melanoma is almost always curable by surgical excision alone. Melanomas that infiltrate into the dermis are considered to be in a "vertical" growth phase and have metastatic or "tumorigenic" potential. Nodular melanomas have no identifiable radial growth or in situ phase and appear to enter the vertical growth phase from their inception, resulting in thicker tumors at diagnosis.

In order to determine the stage of melanoma and, consequently, the physician's tactics and therapy regimen, it is common to use the levels of Clarke's invasion (1969), as well as the international TNM system. The level of invasion by Clark allows you to determine the number of layers of the epidermis affected by melanoma at the time of its detection. The system for determining the level of invasion according to Clark is historically the first system for determining the stage of invasion of melanoma into the epidermis, according to which tumors are divided into five stages (**Table 1**).

The depth of invasion is determined by the stages of Breslow (1970) [12]:

- Thin: the depth of invasion is less than 0.75 mm.

- Intermediate: the depth of invasion is 0.76–3.99 mm.

- Thick (deep): the depth of invasion is more than 4 mm.

After establishing the categories T, N, and M, they are grouped to determine the stage of the disease, which is expressed in Roman numerals from I to IV.

Stage 0: melanoma in situ (Clark level I), 99.9% survival rate
Stage I/II: invasive melanoma, survival rate of 89–95%
T1a: primary tumor thickness less than 1.0 mm, without ulceration $<1/mm^2$
T1b: primary tumor thickness less than 1.0 mm, with ulceration $\geq1/mm^2$
T2a: thickness of the primary tumor 1.01–2.0 mm, without ulceration.
Stage II: high-risk melanoma, 45–79% survival
T2b: primary tumor thickness 1.01–2.0 mm, with ulceration
T3a: primary tumor thickness 2.01–4.0 mm, without ulceration
T3b: primary tumor thickness 2.01–4.0 mm, with ulceration
T4a: thickness of the primary tumor is more than 4.0 mm, without ulcerationT4b: thickness of the primary tumor is more than 4.0 mm, with ulceration.
Stage III: regional metastases, survival 24–70%
N1: single lymph node affected
N2: from two to three affected lymph nodes or regional metastases of the skin
N3: four affected lymph nodes or one lymph node with regional skin metastases.
Stage IV: distant metastases, survival rate of 7–19%
M1a: distant skin metastases, normal LDH.
M1b: lung metastases, normal LDH.
M1c: other distant metastases or any distant metastases with elevated LDH [6, 8].

The American Joint Committee on Cancer recently published its eighth edition of staging criteria, which went into effect as of 1 January, 2018. The impact of Breslow depth and mitoses has been adjusted in the new AJCC staging. The most significant change is that all tumors with a Breslow depth of 0.8–1.0 mm are now staged as T1b. Non-ulcerated tumors with a Breslow depth of <0.7 mm are still

Clark stage	Characteristics	Patient survival
The level of invasion I	All tumor cells are in the epidermis and do not reach the basal membrane	98–100%
The level of invasion II	Tumor cells infiltrate the papillary layer of the dermis	72–96%
The level of invasion III	The tumor reaches the border between the papillary and reticular dermis. The tumor enters the phase of vertical growth	46–90%
The level of invasion IV	Tumor cells are detected in the reticular layer of the dermis	31–67%
The level of invasion V	The tumor invades in the fatty tissue	12–48%

Table 1.
Microscopic melanomas by Clark (1969) [7].

classified as T1a. In addition, Breslow depth is now reported to the nearest 10th decimal place. Therefore, with rounding, T1b tumors encompass 0.75–1.04 mm or any ulcerated tumor of <0.7 mm [8]. Mitoses are no longer part of the criteria to upstage from T1a to T1b. There were no changes to T2–T4 staging. The clinical stage groups were not altered; T1a is still stage 1A, and T1b is still stage 1B [8].

4. Etiopathogenesis

One of the theories supporting the possible effect of pregnancy on tumor transformation is that pregnancy is considered a state of immunodeficiency, necessary to prevent the development of an immune response to fetal antigens. Although the exact mechanism by which tolerance to the fetus development is unclear, several immunological changes may allow the fetus to develop and grow. During pregnancy, the level of granulocytes increases, the number of monocytes remains unchanged, and a significant decrease in lymphocytes is also observed. T-lymphocyte activity is suppressed, and a disruption in the production of interleukins and interferon-G is demonstrated. However, the function of B-lymphocytes remains unchanged, and therefore the immune system during pregnancy is described as a bias toward the humoral immunity, which is more responsible for the formation of antibodies. This change in the balance of Th1 and Th2 cells is similar to the immunological state of patients with oncology [6]. Another possible mechanism of fetal tolerance involves the secretion of protein B7-H1 (CD274) by trophoblast cells; the B7-H1 protein induces apoptosis of activated T cells. This is important because it is also reported that melanoma can elude immune surveillance and secrete B7-H1. The combined secretion of B7-H1 can lead to the fact that melanoma during pregnancy grows and metastasizes more quickly. In addition, it was found that human leukocyte antigen HLA-G is expressed by placental trophoblast cells. Recent studies have shown the role of mutations BRAF V600E in 50% of all skin melanoma development [9]. The fact is that under the influence of excessive UV irradiation, there is a V600 mutation consisting of replacing valine with leucine (V600L), lysine (V600K), or glutamic acid (V600E) in the 600th position, which serves as a signal for the onset of neoplastic transformation. An important role in determining the prognosis is also the age and gender of the patient (women have a better prognosis), tumor localization, lymph node involvement, and the presence of tumor suppressor genes

(CDKN2A, CDK4) and proliferative markers (PCNA, Ki-67) and the presence of thromboses and thromboembolism. Thrombotic complications are the most common complications of paraneoplastic syndrome, manifested by arterial and venous thrombotic occlusions, migrating thrombophlebitis, pulmonary embolism, palpable non-bacterial thromboendocarditis, paradoxical bleeding, and thrombotic microangiopathy. Clinically, venous thromboembolism and malignant neoplasm have two main manifestations: firstly, thrombosis can be the only clinical manifestation of the tumor process, and secondly, in patients with cancer at all stages of the disease, thrombosis may develop [7, 10, 11]. Approximately 10% of melanomas are familial. Among subjects from melanoma families, defined as kindreds in which melanoma occurred in two or more blood relatives, the likelihood of developing melanoma is even greater among those family members who have dysplastic nevi. In a subset of these kindreds, the apparent familial pattern of inheritance may be attributable to clustering of sporadic cases in families who share common heavy sun exposure and susceptible skin type, making genetic analysis and risk stratification more challenging. This concept is substantiated by studies in which *CDKN2A* mutation status, sun exposure, and prevalence of dysplastic/benign nevi influence melanoma risk in families unselected for family history as well as melanoma-prone families.

5. Factors of the risk and clinical picture

The clinical recognition of melanoma, and in particular of early melanoma, may be challenging, even for the most experienced dermatologist. It has been estimated that the sensitivity of the clinical diagnosis of experienced dermatologists is approximately 70% [13]. However, the use of diagnostic aids such as dermoscopy, which requires some training, may greatly improve the sensitivity and specificity of the clinical diagnosis [14].

5.1 History and risk factors

Key questions that should be asked to patients presenting with a lesion that is of concern or for a general examination of their nevi include:

- When was the lesion (or a change in a preexisting lesion) first noticed?

- Does the patient have a personal or family history of melanoma or other skin cancers?

- Does the patient have a history of excessive sun exposure and/or tanning bed use?

- Did the patient suffer severe sunburns during childhood or teenage years?

- Does the patient have a cancer-prone syndrome (e.g., familial atypical multiple mole-melanoma syndrome or xeroderma pigmentosum)?

- Is the patient immunosuppressed?

- Did the patient receive prolonged psoralen plus ultraviolet A (PUVA) therapy?

The patient's phenotypic features associated with an increased risk of melanoma should also be assessed. They include:

- fair-complexioned phototype

- red or blond hair

- light eye color

- presence of a large number (>50) of melanocytic nevi (common nevi)

- presence of atypical melanocytic nevi (benign nevi that clinically share some of the clinical features of melanoma, such as large diameter, irregular borders, and multiple colors)

Clinicians assess the probability that a pigmented lesion is a melanoma using a complex cognitive process that includes a combination of the following steps: visual analysis and pattern recognition, comparative analysis of nevus patterns in an individual patient, and dynamic analysis:

- Visual analysis and pattern recognition typically assess whether a given pigmented lesion has one or more features that may suggest melanoma, including asymmetry, irregular borders, variegated color, and diameter > 6 mm. These features have been included in the widely adopted ABCDE checklist: **A**symmetry (if a lesion is bisected, one half is not identical to the other half), **B**order irregularities, **C**olor variegation (the presence of multiple shades of red, blue, black, gray, or white), **D**iameter ≥ 6 mm, and **E**volution (a lesion that is changing in size, shape, or color or a new lesion, a clinical prediction rule that was devised to help clinicians and laypeople identify suspicious lesions).

- The intrapatient comparative analysis uses the so-called "ugly duckling" sign, which refers to the presence of a single lesion that does not match the patient's nevus phenotype (the so-called signature nevus).

- A history of change in size, color, or shape of a preexisting melanocytic lesion (the "E" for "evolution" in the ABCDE checklist) is the most important clinical criterion for the diagnosis of melanoma. A change can be noted by the patient or documented by comparison of serial clinical or dermoscopic images.

6. Management of melanoma during pregnancy

The evaluation and management of the pregnant woman are similar to that of the nonpregnant woman and are based upon the stage of disease. However, there are potential concerns that arise even in the initial biopsy of suspected melanoma. As the stage of disease becomes more advanced, evaluation and management decisions become more complex in order to ensure safety of the mother and the fetus [1, 2].

A changing pigmented lesion during pregnancy that is clinically and dermatoscopically of concern as a possible melanoma should be biopsied immediately, as it would be in a nonpregnant patient. Excisional biopsy is the optimal way to evaluate a primary cutaneous melanoma. If the pregnant patient is considered a candidate for sentinel lymph node biopsy, there is controversy about the technique and timing of the procedure. In the case of a woman with advanced melanoma, imaging studies may be considered. According to a Committee Opinion Summary published by the American College of Obstetrics and Gynecologists' Committee on Obstetric

Practice, chest radiograph with appropriate shielding, ultrasonography, and magnetic resonance imaging (MRI; preferably without gadolinium) are the techniques of choice for imaging of the pregnant female [15]. In addition, studies such as other radiography, computed tomography (CT) scan (without contrast), and nuclear medicine imaging studies can be utilized since they are typically administered at doses that do not lead to fetal harm.

Some studies have suggested that melanomas diagnosed during pregnancy are more often of greater Breslow depth [16], but a larger proportion of studies have not observed a significant difference. Likewise, a retrospective review analyzed both clinical and pathologic characteristics of 34 melanomas diagnosed during pregnancy and up to 1 year after delivery and compared these with melanomas from age- and disease-matched controls. There was no significant difference in Breslow depth, ulceration, mitotic rate, stage of disease, anatomic location of the primary tumor, histologic subtype, Clark level, regression, necrosis, or vascular invasion [2].

While melanoma is the most common cancer to metastasize to the fetus, metastasis across the placenta to the fetus is rare and is only observed in women with widely metastatic disease [17–19] (**Figure 1**). Even if placental involvement with melanoma is identified, it has been estimated that the fetus is affected in only 25% of these cases. In cases of maternal advanced disease, it is important to alert the pathologist to perform meticulous sectioning of the placenta since many sections may be needed to detect small foci of melanoma.

The general approach to the treatment of pregnancy-associated melanoma is based upon the same prognostic factors as for nonpregnant woman. Melanoma diagnosed during pregnancy is a rare clinical case presentation which must be mastered. In the absence of guidelines for this clinical challenge, we performed a review of the literature and provide a practical guideline on how to manage such rare clinical cases based on our clinical experience. Expecting mothers require adequate counseling and explanation of all therapeutic options as they take responsibility for more than their own lives. However, they should be guided through the process of diagnostic and therapeutic measures in a potentially life-threatening situation. Pregnancy itself is no reason to withhold any type of necessary melanoma surgery. Perioperative management, however, requires certain adjustments in order to comply with this special situation. If indicated, even adjuvant and palliative systemic therapies need to be given to the patient, but they also have to be adapted to the specific circumstances as data is still sparse, especially for the new first- and second-line therapies with antibodies and targeted molecules.

Management becomes more complex once the need for SLNB is established or if the patient has more advanced disease and should be individualized. In advanced melanoma, the newest agents, such as BRAF inhibitors (vemurafenib and dabrafenib) and checkpoint inhibitors [nivolumab and ipilimumab (anti-programed cell death-1 and anti-CTLA, respectively)], may be teratogenic [17–21]. The FDA-approved patient labeling recommends avoidance of pregnancy and lactation during BRAF inhibitor therapy and up to 2 weeks after the last dose, during ipilimumab therapy and up to 3 months after the last dose, and during nivolumab therapy and up to 5 months after the last dose.

The patient with a thin melanoma with excellent prognosis need not delay future pregnancies or avoid the use of oral contraceptives or hormone replacement therapy, if the latter are indicated.

The combination of pregnancy and the high stage of melanoma are a dangerous condition requiring careful risk assessment by the obstetrician-gynecologist and oncologist. Earlier, women with melanoma III and IV stages were artificially interrupted by pregnancy according to medical indications. However, at present, in relation to risk stratification and pregnancy management in women with melanoma associated with pregnancy, there is a view that therapeutic approaches are almost the same as those of nonpregnant ones and are determined by the stage of the disease. For patients with a history of melanoma and multiple dysplastic nevi, a more frequent dermatological examination during pregnancy is suggested. With regard to recommendations for the implementation of the reproductive function, it is shown that a future pregnancy should not be delayed in a woman with a thin localized melanoma with a favorable prognosis. For patients with progressive

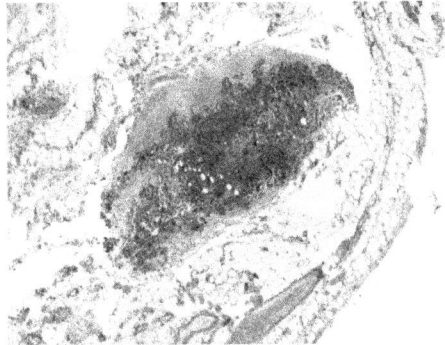

(a)

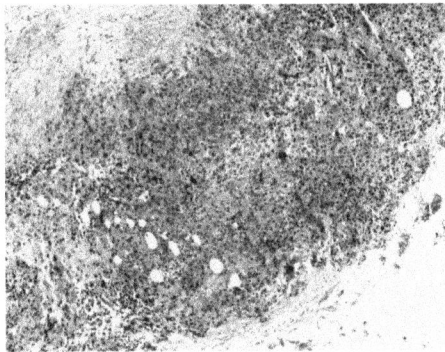

(b)

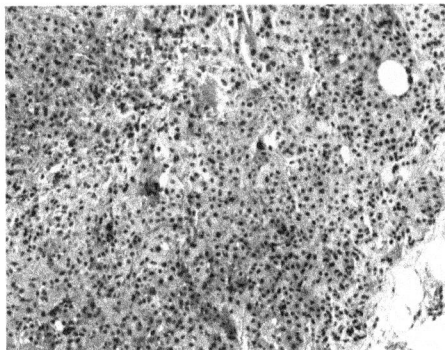

(c)

Figure 1.
Histological examination of biopsy (intraoperative) material (hematoxylin-eosin staining). The material is represented by a lymph node located among adipose tissue with tumor metastasis (a), which has the structure of epithelioid cell melanoma with a high content of pigment (b). The tumor totally replaces the tissue of the lymph node with the germination of the capsule (c).

disease, it is recommended to wait at least 2–3 years before pregnancy, since during this time interval relapses are most likely [13, 15, 22]. However, this issue should be considered individually in each specific observation, since a woman of late reproductive age may be concerned about the implementation of reproduction in the event of a pregnancy failure. The problem becomes even more controversial in a woman with a common form of the disease, because her life expectancy remains unclear. Decision-making becomes much more complex in the woman with a more uncertain prognosis where a delay in future pregnancy may be considered, but this should be evaluated on a case-by-case basis.

Author details

Ignatko Irina Vladimirovna* and Strizhakov Alexander Nikolaevich
Federal State Autonomous Educational Institution of Higher Education
I.M. Sechenov First Moscow State Medical University of the Ministry of Health of the Russian Federation, Sechenov University, Moscow, Russia

*Address all correspondence to: iradocent@mail.ru

IntechOpen

References

[1] Jhaveri MB, Driscoll MS, Grant-Kels JM. Melanoma in pregnancy. Clinical Obstetrics and Gynecology. 2011;**54**(4):537-545. DOI: 10.1097/GRF.0b013e318236e18b

[2] Driscoll MS, Stein JA, Grant-Kels JM. Melanoma in pregnancy. UpToDate. 2016

[3] Andersson TM, Johansson AL, Fredriksson I, Lambe M. Cancer during pregnancy and the postpartum period: A population-based study. Cancer. 2015;**121**(12):2072-2077

[4] Pack GT, Scharnagel IM. The prognosis for malignant melanoma in the pregnant woman. Cancer. 1951;**4**(2):324

[5] Ribero S, Longo C, Dika E, Fortes C, Pasquali S, Nagore E, et al. Pregnancy and melanoma: A European-wide survey to assess current management and a critical literature overview. Journal of the European Academy of Dermatology and Venereology. 2017;**31**(1):65

[6] Lens MB, Rosdahl I, Ahlbom A, Farahmand BY, Synnerstad I, Boeryd B, et al. Effect of pregnancy on survival in women with cutaneous malignant melanoma. Journal of Clinical Oncology. 2004;**22**(21):4369

[7] Lattanzi M, Lee Y, Simpson D, Moran U, Darvishian F, Kim RH, et al. Primary melanoma histologic subtype: Impact on survival and response to therapy. Journal of the National Cancer Institute. 2019;**111**(2):180

[8] Chiaravalloti AJ, Jinna S, Kerr PE, Whalen J, Grant-Kels JM. A deep look into thin melanomas: What's new for the clinician and the impact on the patient. International Journal of Women's Dermatology. 2018;**4**(3):119-121. DOI: 10.1016/j.ijwd.2018.01.003. ISSN: 2352-6475

[9] Johansson AL, Andersson TM, Plym A, Ullenhag GJ, Møller H, Lambe M. Mortality in women with pregnancy-associated malignant melanoma. Journal of the American Academy of Dermatology. 2014;**71**(6):1093-1101. Epub: October 16, 2014

[10] Tellez A, Rueda S, Conic RZ, Powers K, Galdyn I, Mesinkovska NA, et al. Risk factors and outcomes of cutaneous melanoma in women less than 50 years of age. Journal of the American Academy of Dermatology. 2016;**74**(4):731

[11] Møller H, Purushotham A, Linklater KM, Garmo H, Holmberg L, Lambe M, et al. Recent childbirth is an adverse prognostic factor in breast cancer and melanoma, but not in Hodgkin lymphoma. European Journal of Cancer. 2013;**49**(17):3686-3693. Epub: August 6, 2013

[12] Gachon J, Beaulieu P, Sei JF, Gouvernet J, Claudel JP, Lemaitre M, et al. First prospective study of the recognition process of melanoma in dermatological practice. Archives of Dermatology. 2005;**141**(4):434

[13] Brady MS, Noce NS. Pregnancy is not detrimental to the melanoma patient with clinically localized disease. The Journal of Clinical and Aesthetic Dermatology. 2010;**3**:22-28

[14] Vestergaard ME, Macaskill P, Holt PE, Menzies SW. Dermoscopy compared with naked eye examination for the diagnosis of primary melanoma: A meta-analysis of studies performed in a clinical setting. The British Journal of Dermatology. 2008;**159**(3):669

[15] Stensheim H, Møller B, van Dijk T, Fosså SD. Cause-specific survival for women diagnosed with cancer during pregnancy or lactation: A registry-based cohort study. Journal of Clinical Oncology. 2009;**27**(1):45

[16] Baergen RN, Johnson D, Moore T, Benirschke K. Maternal melanoma metastatic to the placenta: A case report and review of the literature. Archives of Pathology & Laboratory Medicine. 1997;**121**(5):508

[17] Ignatko IV, Strizhakov AN, Protsenko DN, Afanasjeva NV, Djadykov IN, Zairatyantz GO, et al. Melanoma and pregnancy: Risks, course and prognosis. Gynecology, Obstetrics and Perinatology. 2018;**17**(1):83-87. DOI: 10.20953/1726-1678-2018-1-83-87

[18] Fedorenko IV, Paraiso KHT, Smalley KSM. Acquired and intrinsic BRAF inhibitor resistance in BRAF V600E mutant melanoma. Biochemical Pharmacology. 2011;**82**(3):201-209

[19] Driscoll MS, Grant-Kels JM. Hormones, nevi, and melanoma: An approach to the patient. Journal of the American Academy of Dermatology. 2007;**57**(6):919

[20] Vorobiev AV, Makatsaria AD, Bitsadze VO, Brenner B. Dysfunction of the hemostatic system and carcinogenesis: The current state of the matter. Obstetrics and Gynecology. 2017;**8**:28-33. DOI: 10.18565/aig.2017.8.28-33

[21] Chapman PB, Robert C, Larkin J, Haanen JB. Vemurafenib in patients with BRAFV600 mutation-positive metastatic melanoma: Final overall survival results of the randomized BRIM-3 study. Annals of Oncology. 2017;**28**(10):2581-2587. DOI: 10.1093/annonc/mdx339

[22] Committee Opinion No. 656. Guidelines for diagnostic imaging during pregnancy and lactation: American College of Obstetricians and Gynecologists' Committee on Obstetric Practice. Obstetrics and Gynecology. 2016;**127**(2):e75-e80

Chapter 5

Subungual Melanoma

Mariana Catalina De Anda Juárez

Abstract

Subungual melanoma (SUM) is a subtype of acral melanoma. Its incidence in dark phototypes, Hispanics and Asians, is around 20% and accounts for 50% of acral melanomas. It is an infrequent subtype in Caucasians representing only 3%. Subungual melanoma arises from dormant melanocytes in the nail matrix and exceptionally from melanocytes in the nail bed. In its initial phases of radial growth, it presents as longitudinal melanonychia. The differential diagnoses are melanocytic activation (racial, traumatic), nail matrix nevi, and lentigos. Prognosis depends on Breslow depth at diagnosis. For in situ melanoma, treatment consists of conservative surgical removal of the nail unit with 5 mm margins.

Keywords: subungual melanoma, longitudinal melanonychia, acral melanoma, nail melanoma

1. Introduction

Subungual melanoma (SUM) is a subtype of acral lentiginous melanoma. It is a rare subtype in Caucasians accounting for 3% of all melanomas. In dark phototypes, Hispanics and Asians, it represents 20%, and it is the most frequent malignancy of the nail unit [1].

SUM or nail melanoma arises from dormant melanocytes in the nail unit, mainly in the nail matrix, and exceptionally in the nail bed.

UV radiation is not considered an important risk factor for this subtype of melanoma. Trauma has been a hypothetical etiologic agent. Many patients associate direct trauma to the onset of this malignancy, and it has been hypothesized that inflammation can cause mutations in melanocytes during trauma-induced proliferation; but a direct association has not been proven, and it may only be a coincidence due to increased attention to a longitudinal melanonychia after trauma [2].

SUM has a long radial growth phase that can last for many years; in this stage it presents as longitudinal melanonychia, and the differential diagnosis includes racial and traumatic melanocytic activation, nail matrix nevi, and lentigo of the nail unit [3].

Nail plate pigmentation can also be caused by blood and external pigments such as silver in argyria. Many drugs cause nail pigmentation by drug deposition or by melanocytic activation (minocycline, psoralens, cyclophosphamide, zidovudine). Bacterial or fungal infections (*Proteus mirabilis*, *Aspergillus* sp., *Candida* sp., *Trichophyton rubrum*) can cause nail pigmentation; other subungual tumors such as epidermoid carcinoma and even a subungual wart can present as longitudinal melanonychia [3].

Clues to the diagnosis of melanoma include a single-digit affection, melanonychia wider than 3 mm with a triangular form (this means that the band is growing), rapid widening of a longitudinal melanonychia, onset in adulthood (melanoma in children is quite rare), and Hutchinson's and micro-Hutchinson's sign [4] (**Figure 1** and **Table 1**).

In more advanced stages, SUM causes nail dystrophy, ridging, partial destruction of the nail plate, ulceration, bleeding, and total destruction of the nail unit (**Figure 2**).

SUM affects women and men equally, although some series report a slight predominance in women. SUM is more common on the dominant hand, and it is more frequently reported on the thumbs and on the first finger on both toes [1].

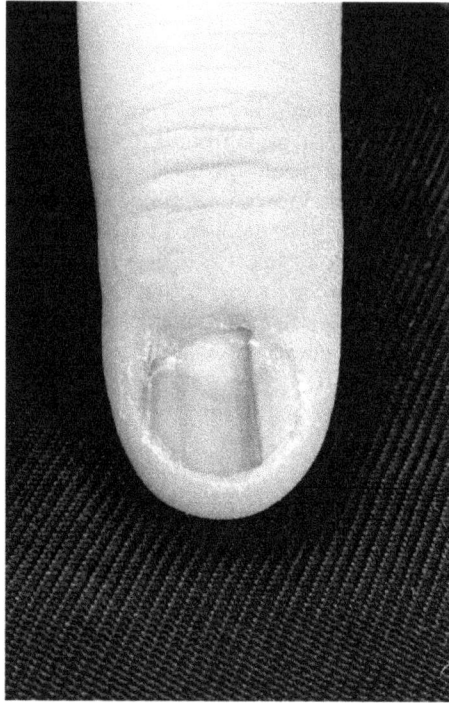

Figure 1.
SUM in situ. Longitudinal irregular melanonychia with nail plate ridging.

A	Age: 40–60 years. Does not rule out in children African, American, Asian, Hispanics
B	Band: brown-black irregular Blurred borders >4 mm
C	Change: rapid increase in size No change: failure to improve
D	Single digit: Thumb-hallux-index finger Dominant hand Nail dystrophy: ridging ulceration
E	Extension—Hutchinson's sign: pigment on nail folds Micro-Hutchinson: cuticle pigmentation visible with dermoscopy
F	Family or personal history of melanoma
Adapted from [4].	

Table 1. *ABC rule to suspect SUM.*

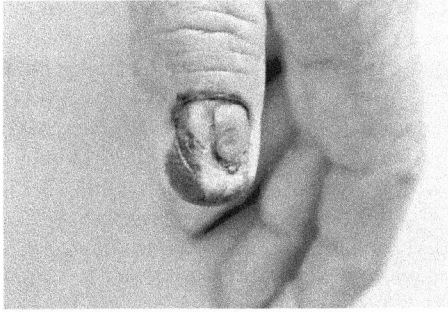

Figure 2.
Invasive SUM with Hutchinson's sign and partial destruction of the nail plate.

SUM is frequently diagnosed in advanced stages, due to a delay in diagnosis by healthcare providers not aware of its existence and clinical presentation or due to lack of access to medical services. The median Breslow at diagnosis is between 4 and 6 mm [1].

2. Dermoscopy

Dermoscopy of the nail unit is a noninvasive method that can help identify high-risk features.

Dermoscopy is useful to distinguish blood; subungual hemorrhage has a distinctive pattern of globules with distal streaks, a filamentous end, and red to brown or deep purple color. It is important to consider a bleeding tumor and rule out that possibility [5].

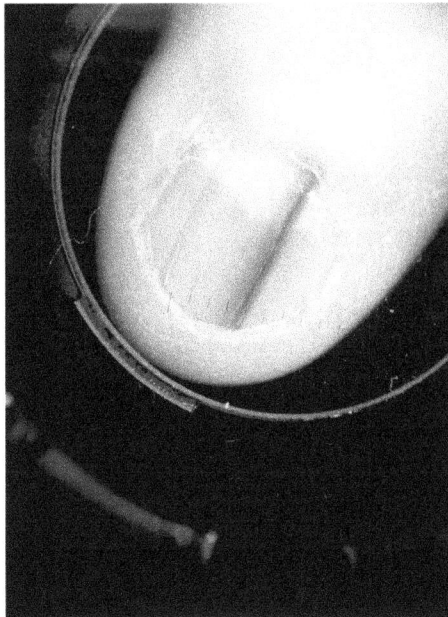

Figure 3.
Dermoscopy of SUM in situ. Irregular multiple heterogenous brown bands with blurred edges and microhutchinson's sign.

Subungual melanoma should be suspected and ruled out in heterogeneous longitudinal brown or black melanonychias, when bands are irregular in color, thickness, and spacing. SUM can also present as a diffuse dark background with barely visible lines (**Figure 3**). When a brown coloration in the background is overlaid by regular, parallel, and pigmented lines, the most probable diagnosis is a nevus.

Edge blurring is another sign associated with SUM. Hutchinson's sign is considered an indicator of SUM; however, it can also be found in benign nevi. Atypical Hutchinson's sign in SUM is asymmetric and polychromatic, and the pigment is distributed in a disorderly fashion. Micro-Hutchinson's sign is periungual pigmentation invisible to the naked eye and only observed with dermoscopy; it has only been described in SUM. Triangular shape of the longitudinal band (wider proximally than distally) indicates rapid growth [5, 6].

A grayish longitudinal background either alone or overlaid by thin homogenous gray lines is suggestive of melanocytic hyperplasia as in lentigo or lentiginoses (Laugier-Hunziker syndrome, Leopard syndrome, Peutz-Jeghers-Touraine disease), in drug-induced, ethnic, and traumatic nail pigmentation.

Amelanotic SUM is a very difficult diagnosis; in this rare case, the nail plate is often partially destroyed by a bleeding, erythematous vegetating tumor. Dermoscopy can show areas of remanant pigmentation and vascular disorder: irregular vessels and milky-red areas [5].

3. Nail matrix biopsy

Nail matrix biopsy remains essential for diagnosis. Most melanomas arise from the distal matrix; by performing dermoscopy of the free edge of the nail plate, it is sometimes possible to determine the origin of melanonychia. If the distal matrix is the origin of melanonychia, the ventral aspect of the nail plate will be affected, and if the proximal nail matrix is the origin, the dorsal aspect of the nail plate will be pigmented.

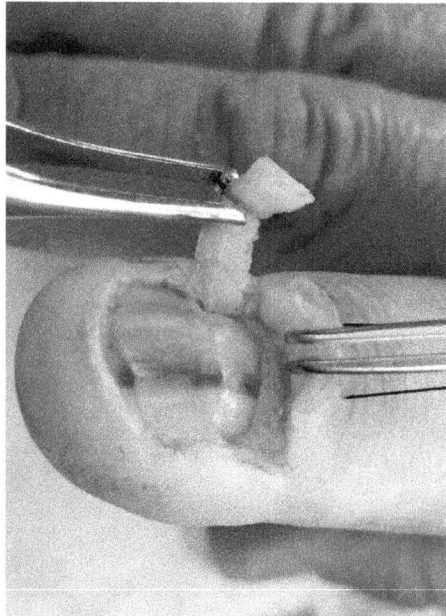

Figure 4.
Nail matrix biopsy technique: proximal nail fold flap and exposure of the nail matrix.

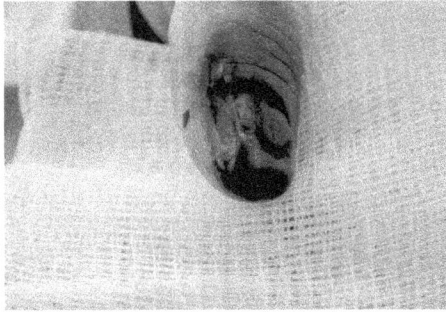

Figure 5.
Lateral longitudinal nail biopsy.

The surgical technique consists in exposing the nail matrix, identifying the origin of melanonychia, and taking a representative sample of the nail matrix without leaving permanent nail dystrophy. This technique is performed under digital block anesthesia. First, the nail plate has to be removed, and a flap of the proximal nail fold elevated so that the proximal and distal nail matrix is exposed (**Figure 4**).

Intraoperative dermoscopy of the nail matrix is an effective tool to precisely identify the origin of the pigment. A longitudinal matrix biopsy, no more than 3-mm-wide or a 3-mm-punch biopsy, can be done without risk of dystrophy; a shave biopsy of the matrix 1 mm deep is enough to make the diagnosis and lessens the risk of permanent dystrophy. There is no need to suture the nail matrix; the nail plate and the proximal nail fold are relocated and sutured with a 4-0 nonabsorbable suture.

In cases of invasive SUM, a lateral longitudinal nail biopsy that includes the proximal fold, the matrix lateral horn, the nail bed, the plate, and the distal nail fold is easier to perform and gives the pathologist enough tissue to make the diagnosis and report Breslow depth (**Figure 5**).

4. Histology

Nail matrix biopsy is still essential for SUM diagnosis. Normal nail matrix has between 4 and 14 melanocytes per mm (mean 6.86 cells/mm per mm stretch of nail matrix epithelium) [7].

The presence of nests without atypia is distinctive of nevi, especially in a child with a well-demarcated, uniformly pigmented, single, longitudinal band [8].

The histologic distinction between a benign subungual pigmented macule (lentigo or lentigo-like hyperpigmentation) and an early lesion of SUM can be difficult.

This benign lentigos may histologically only show an increase in melanin deposition in keratinocytes, melanocytes, and/or macrophages without proliferation of melanocytes (melanocytic activation). However, these benign lesions may show proliferation of melanocytes as well. The mean density of melanocytes in lentigos is around 15.3 cells per 1-mm-stretch nail matrix. There is no confluence of melanocytes. Cytologic atypia has to be absent or mild. There is no inflammation associated. Pagetoid spread may be present but only focally.

SUM in situ shows a much greater proliferation of melanocytes (mean 58.9 cells per 1 mm of stretched nail matrix) that ranges from 39 to 136 melanocytes per 1 mm of stretched nail matrix. There is at least focal confluence of cells with various grades of cytologic atypia: nuclear enlargement, hyperchromatism, irregular nuclear contours, and prominent nucleolus. Dendrites are thicker and larger. Pagetoid spread is found in almost all lesions of SUM, and inflammation in the epithelial stromal interface is frequent [6, 7]. In some cases of SUM with lentigi-nous growth of single atypical melanocytes, immunohistochemical stains with MELAN-A and HMB-45 may ease the diagnosis.

Invasive SUM has denser proliferation of atypical melanocytes arranged in aggregates and sheaths and may lead to nail dystrophy, nail destruction, and ulceration.

It can be difficult to measure Clark level and Breslow thickness, because the distinction of the onychodermis is not always clear and the underlying phalanx is separated by only a thin dermal collagen layer [6].

5. Treatment

SUM in situ must be surgically removed with wide resection of the entire nail unit with a 5-mm-wide margin and periosteum depth (**Figure 6**).

Reconstruction can be performed with the next finger banner flap and a full thickness graft, or it heals by the second intention with good functional results [1].

Treatment for invasive SUM is amputation of the phalanx.

Sentinel lymph node biopsy should be performed in SUM with Breslow depth >1 mm and in SUM >0.8 mm with ulceration [1, 9–11].

The most important factors for prognosis and survival are Breslow depth, ulceration, and nodal status at diagnosis [10, 11].

SUM has the same prognostic factors as other subtypes of melanoma. The adverse outcomes associated with SUM are due to delay in diagnosis because of a lack in recognition by health professionals and advanced stages at diagnosis.

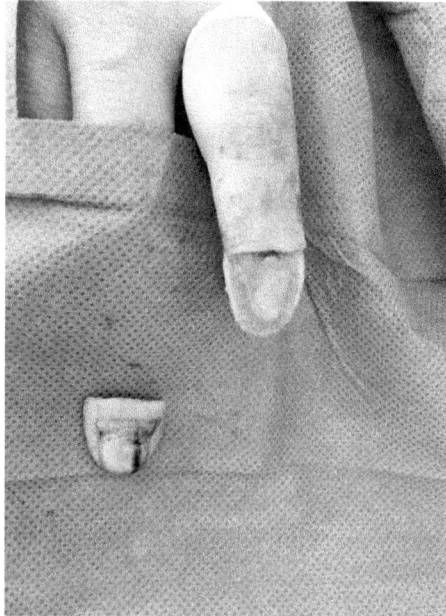

Figure 6.
Resection of the nail unit with 5 mm wide margins and periosteum depth.

Author details

Mariana Catalina De Anda Juárez
Department of Dermatology and Dermatologic surgery, "Dr. Manuel Gea
González" General Hospital, Mexico City, Mexico

*Address all correspondence to: mdeanda73@gmail.com

IntechOpen

References

[1] Anda-Juárez MC, Martínez-Velasco MA, Fonte-Ávalos V, Toussaint-Caire S, Domínguez-Cherit J. Conservative surgical management of in situ subungual melanoma: Long-term follow-up. Anais Brasileiros de Dermatologia. 2016;**91**(6):846-848

[2] Möhrle M, Häfner HM. Is subungual melanoma related to trauma? Dermatology. 2002;**204**(4):259-261

[3] Dominguez-Cherit J, Roldan-Marin R, Pichardo-Velazquez P, Valente C, Fonte-Avalos V, Vega-Memije ME, et al. Melanocytic hyperplasia, and nail melanoma in a Hispanic population. Journal of the American Academy of Dermatology. 2008;**59**(5):785-791

[4] Levit EK, Kagen MH, Scher RK, Grossman M, Altman E. The ABC rule for clinical detection of subungual melanoma. Journal of the American Academy of Dermatology. 2000;**42**(2 Pt 1):269-274

[5] Luc T, Dalle S. Dermoscopy provides useful information for the management of melanonychia striata. Dermatologic Therapy. 2007;**20**:3-10

[6] Domínguez-Cherit J, Gutiérrez-Mendoza D, de Anda-Juarez M. Subungual melanoma. In: Di Chiacchio N, Tosti A, editors. Melanonychias. Switzerland: Springer International Publishing; 2017. pp. 71-84. DOI: 10.1007/978-3-319-44993-7.ch7

[7] Perrin C, Michelis JF, Boyer J, Ambrosetti D. Melanocytes pattern in the normal nail, with special reference to nail bed melanocytes. The American Journal of Dermatopathology. Mar 2018;**40**(3):180-184

[8] Amin B, Nehal K, Jungbluth A. Histologic distinction between subungual lentigo and melanoma. The American Journal of Surgical Pathology. 2008;**32**:835-843

[9] Mannava K, Mannava S, Koman L. Longitudinal melanonychia: Detection and management of nail melanoma. Hand Surgery. 2013;**18**(1):133-139

[10] Coit DG, Thompson JA, Albertini MR, et al. Cutaneous Melanoma, Version 2.2019, NCCN Clinical Practice Guidelines in Oncology. Journal of the National Comprehensive Cancer Network. 1 Apr 2019;**17**(4):367-402. DOI: 10.6004/jnccn.2019.0018

[11] Gershenwald J, Scolyer R. Melanoma staging: American Joint Committee on Cancer (AJCC) 8th edition and beyond. Annals of Surgical Oncology. 2018;**25**:2105-2110

Mathematic Models for Tumor Detection

Chapter 6

2D Fourier Fractal Analysis of Optical Coherence Tomography Images of Basal Cell Carcinomas and Melanomas

Wei Gao, Bingjiang Lin, Valery P. Zakharov and Oleg O. Myakinin

Abstract

The optical coherence tomography (OCT) technique is applied in the diagnosis of the skin tissue. In general, quantitative imaging features obtained from OCT images have already been used as biomarkers to categorize skin tumors. Particularly, the fractal dimension (FD) could be capable of providing an efficient approach for analyzing OCT images of skin tumors. The 2D Fourier fractal analysis (FFA) as well as the differential box counting method (DBCM) was used in this paper to classify the basal cell carcinomas (BCC), melanomas, and benign melanocytic nevi. Generalized estimating equations were used to test for differences between skin tumors. Our results showed that the significant decrease of the 2D FD was detected in the benign melanocytic nevi and basal cell carcinomas as compared with the melanomas. Our results also suggested that the 2D FFA could provide a more efficient way to calculating FD to differentiate the basal cell carcinomas, melanomas, and benign melanocytic nevi as compared to the 2D DBCM.

Keywords: skin tumor, basal cell carcinomas, melanomas, fractal dimension, differential box counting method, Fourier fractal analysis, optical coherence tomography

1. Introduction

The OCT technique is an optical imaging modality that could provide high-resolution and cross-sectional visualization of biological tissues [1]. The OCT technique was firstly utilized for imaging retinal tissue [2]. In 1997, the OCT technique was used in the evaluation and the detection of diseases in the skin because it can detect the diseases or wounds in a noninvasive way. The burn wounds and the wound healing processes have been studied by using the OCT technique [3–5]. By utilizing the OCT technique, the morphological changes of skin tissue can be obtained from OCT images. Besides, the OCT technique has been used to analyze the differences in morphological changes in skin tumors [6]. Particularly, the morphological changes can be used as an indicator to characterize the different types of skin tumors.

An automatic texture analysis of OCT images did not have a long history. Gan et al. received accuracy of the atrial tissue disease definition in 80% for OCT imaging, using his own method with automatic detection of regions of interest [7]. Scientists from Stanford offered automatic classifier to determine the basal cell carcinomas by using polarization-sensitive OCT that could achieve the sensitivity and specificity of about 85% [8]. Lingley-Papadopoulos et al. used texture analysis for diseases of the bladder, receiving sensitivity of 92% and specificity of 62% [9]. Gambichler et al. in their work received a sensitivity of about 75% and a specificity of about 93% for the melanomas and nevi in the skin tissue [10]. Multi-beam OCT system has been successfully used to identify the basal cell carcinomas with the sensitivity of 96% and specificity of 75% [11]. The multimodal approach to the problem of separation of intestinal adenocarcinomas from healthy bowel tissue, using texture analysis of OCT images and chemical information Raman spectroscopy, gives the sensitivity and specificity of 94% [12]. Fourier analysis and texture analysis of OCT images of breast tissues ex vivo using Fisher's linear discriminate analysis gives the result as 100% sensitivity and specificity for the normal and pathology case and 90 and 85%, respectively, for the benign/malignant tumors case [13].

Based on the fact that the affected tissue is characterized by the distinct structural changes at the molecular, cellular, and tissue architecture levels, the fractal dimension performed by the fractal analysis can be used to analyze the disease-dependent irregularities in shape. In 1967, Mandelbrot firstly introduced the concept of the fractal dimension to describe the self-similar pattern when he measured the length of the coastline of the United Kingdom [14]. Mandelbrot found that the total length of the coastline changed when he used the different size of ruler to measure the length of coastline. Therefore, he employed the FD as a scale that was applied to the ruler. The scale can be recognized as an indicator to describe the roughness of a surface such as the coastline. And due to this description, the complexity of an object can be evaluated by using the FD. Higher values of the FD mean the higher roughness of the surfaces. Fractal analysis has already been used to study the morphological change of skin tumors.

Hussain et al. used the box counting method to find out the dimensions of the affected cells in skin tumors [15]. Karimi and Farshchi calculated the FD from micros by using the box counting method for differentiating normal moles (nevi) from melanomas [16]. Gao et al. used the 2D DBCM to extract the FD from OCT images for classifying the skin tumors [17]. In those studies, the box counting method (including the DBCM) was applied to the skin tumors' images for extracting the FD.

Though the box counting method is a reasonable methodology to calculate the FD from the skin tumors' images, it is a low-efficient and time-consuming methodology that counts the boxes for calculating FD. In order to improve the efficacy, it is necessary to employ a cheaper and more efficient methodology to extract FD from the images. In this paper, the 2D Fourier fractal methodology was used to reduce the computational time of FD from OCT images. The spectral domain OCT (SD-OCT) was used to collect images for the basal cell carcinomas, melanomas, and benign melanocytic nevi.

2. Methodology

2.1 OCT system and data collection

The SD-OCT equipment was assembled in the department of laser and biotechnical system at the Samara National Research University. The schematic diagram is showed in **Figure 1**. The equipment was characterized by the 14 mW output power, 45 nm light source bandwidth, 840 nm central wavelength, and axial/lateral resolution ca. 6 μm. A Michelson interferometer in the equipment was used to split the incident light in a 50/50 ration for the sample and reference arms. A diffraction grating that could be capable for providing 1200 groves per millimeter and a CCD line scan camera that has the 29.3 kHz line rate in 4096 pixel resolution are assembled in the spectrometer. The image acquisition card for digitizing the signal is NI-IMAQ PCI-1428.

This study included three universities that are the Samara State Medical University, Samara National Research University, and Ningbo University of Technology. The institutional review board of each institution approved the study protocol. This research adhered to the tenets set forth in the Declaration of Helsinki. Informed consent of each subject was obtained.

2.2 OCT images and OCT image processing

The samples of skin tumor with the typical macroscopic features were selected from the surgical removal. Three types of skin tumors were included in this study, which are malignant melanoma, benign melanocytic nevus, and basal cell carcinoma (BCC).

The OCT image of the benign melanocytic nevus obtained by using the SD-OCT was showed in **Figure 2**. The structure of the epidermis in OCT images of benign melanocytic nevus was typical for a healthy skin, although it featured a certain amount of melanocytes and pigmented keratinocytes. As compared to benign melanocytic nevus, basal cell carcinoma and melanoma showed the signs of malignancy that could be used to differentiate themselves from benign melanocytic nevi and normal skin tissue. The OCT image of the basal cell carcinoma was showed in **Figure 3**. The image clearly indicated that the basal cell carcinoma tumor cells were roundish or elliptical in shape. In the periphery of the tumor mass, the basal cell carcinoma cells had palisading arrangement. The optical densities in basal cell carcinoma and normal skin tissue are different, in which the basal cell carcinoma in OCT images showed a darker color. The OCT image of the melanoma was showed in **Figure 4**. In the OCT image, the healthy epidermis can be seen as a bright band on the skin tissue's surface. The melanin complex and the small undifferentiated cells

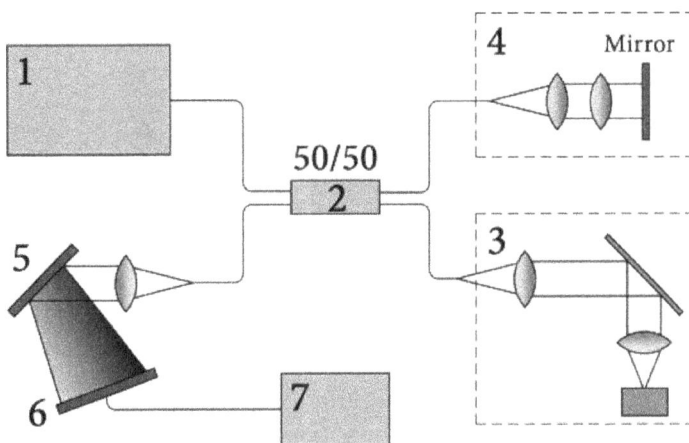

Figure 1.
The custom-built SD-OCT system. (1) Broadband light source, (2) 50/50 beam splitter, (3) sample arm, (4) reference arm, (5) spectrometer with grating, (6) CCD camera, and (7) computer with IMAQ.

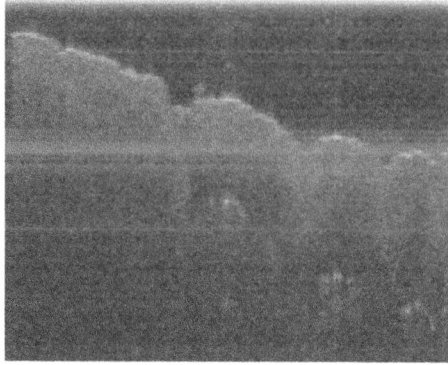

Figure 2.
The OCT image of the benign melanocytic nevi.

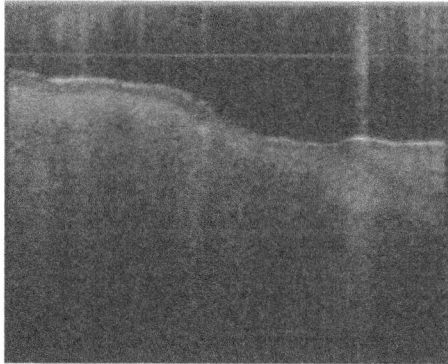

Figure 3.
The OCT image of the basal cell carcinoma.

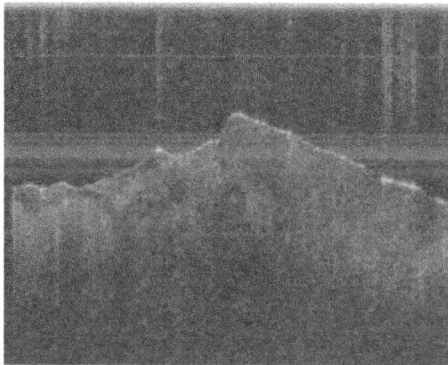

Figure 4.
The OCT image of the melanoma.

without pigment are under the epidermis. Due to the heterogeneity of tumor, the randomly located multiform objects that have the different optical density can be visualized in the OCT images compared to the normal layered structure. The OCT image showed the dark or bright areas since the melanoma cells may have a surplus amount of pigment or may contain the nonpigmented elements.

OCT images were exported from the custom-built OCT system in the form of 8 bit gray level. The structural information of biological tissues can be recorded in OCT images. However, the OCT images contained not only the "useful" information but also the noise. A typical type of noise is called as "speckle" noise. The speckle noise is due to the limited spatial-frequency bandwidth of the interference signals in OCT [18]. Because OCT images were generated from OCT imaging system with the coherent detection, the speckle noise significantly blurred the contrast of OCT images by generating a grainy element in OCT images, which makes it harder to extract the features from OCT images. Therefore, it is necessary to remove the speckle noise from OCT images and then extract the FD to quantitatively classify the skin tumors. In this paper, the interval type II fuzzy anisotropic diffusion filter was employed to remove the speckle noise from OCT images [19].

2.3 Fractal analysis

In Euclidean space, structures consist of basic Euclidean geometries including lines, planes, and cubes. A straight line has exactly one dimension, a plane has exactly two dimensions, and a cube has exactly three dimensions. These basic shapes in integer dimensions were called "topological dimensions." For example, a fractal curve has dimensions between a straight line and a plane (between one and two), and a fractal surface has dimensions between a plane and a cube (between two and three). In order to determine the FD of complex objects, several definitions of FD were used. One simple and easily understandable definition of the FD is the Hausdorff dimension, which can be defined as follows:

$$FD = \lim_{r \to 0} \frac{\log N_r}{\log\left(\frac{1}{r}\right)}, \tag{1}$$

where N_r is the number of sets of cells (i.e., a ruler used to measure the coastline) and $1/r$ is the magnification factor that was used to reduce the cell in each spatial direction.

A typical example of a geometric object with a non-integer dimension is the Koch curve (see **Figure 5**). The straight line A, called the initiator, has a length of 1. The middle third of the line A was replaced with two lines that each line has the same length (1/3) as the remaining lines on each side. Thus, the length of the line B has a length 4/3. This form specifies a rule that is used to generate other new forms. Thus, the curve A was used as the initiator, and the curve B was used as generator for constructing the Koch curve. Each line was replaced with four lines, each 1/3 the length of the original. Therefore, the lengths of the lines C, D, and E are 16/9, 64/27, and 256/81, respectively. As indicated in **Figure 5**, the total length of the curve increases with each step, which leads to an infinite length. By applying Eq. (1), the relationship between $\log N_r$ and $\log(1/r)$ for the Koch curve, the FD could be calculated as $\ln 4/\ln 3 = 1.26$.

Moreover, the measurement of the FD of the coastline could be treated as the Koch curve, which naturally leads to the introduction of the box counting method. In the measurement of the coastline, the number of scaled ruler is also counted as and is the size of the cell (i.e., ruler). Equation (1) is used in the calculation of the FD. Note that the typical cell is a box-shaped cell (a square) for two-dimensional objects and that the typical cell is a cube for three-dimensional objects. The box counting method is considered the most accepted methodology to measure the FD in various applications due to its simplicity and automatic computability [20]. However, the box counting method was pointed to overcount or undercount the number of boxes (cells), which then led to an inaccurate calculation of the

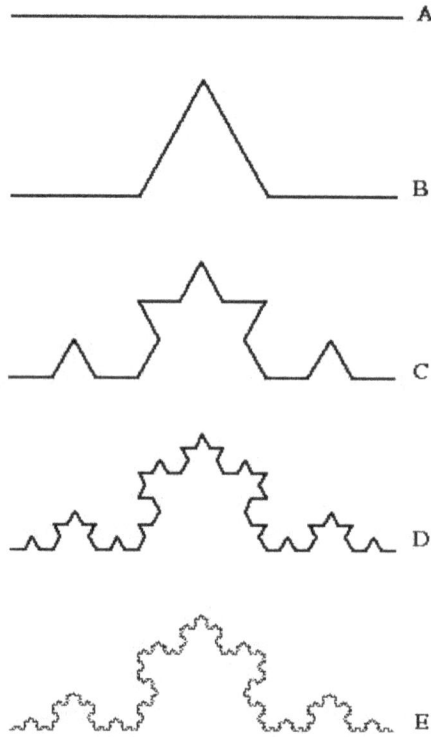

Figure 5.
Koch curve. The initiator (A) and generator (B) are used for constructing the Koch curve. Curves C, D, and E are levels 2, 3, and 4 in the construction of the Koch curve, respectively.

FD. Therefore, a more accurate and robust methodology, the 2D FAA, is utilized for the calculation of the FD.

The method for the calculation of the 2D Fourier FD is applied to a 2D grayscale image $I(k,l)$ with the size $N \times N$. The Fourier transform $\bar{I}$ can be expressed as follows:

$$\bar{I}(u,v) = \sum_{k=0}^{N-1}\sum_{l=0}^{N-1} I(k,l) \exp\left[-\frac{i2\pi}{N}(uk + vl)\right], \qquad (2)$$

where u and v are the horizontal and vertical frequency, respectively. The total frequency f is given by $f = \sqrt{u^2 + v^2}$. Then, the power spectrum of the 2D grayscale image $I(i,j)$ is given by

$$P = cf^{-\beta}, \qquad (3)$$

where c is a constant.

β can be calculated by fitting the function in Eq. (3) by calculating the slope of the curve $lnP \times lnf$. The least square method was used to obtain the slope in this paper. The 2D Fourier FD was then calculated by using the following equation [21]:

$$FD = \frac{8 - \beta}{2}. \qquad (4)$$

The range of possible values is between 2 and 3.

Another methodology the 2D DBCM will be used in this paper to calculate the FD. The detail of the 2D DBCM was introduced in Sarkar's paper [22].

3. Results and discussion

In our previous paper, the quantitative image features including the FD have already been studied to differentiate the skin tumors. However, the FD was extracted from OCT images by using the 2D DBCM. Generally speaking, the 2D DBCM is a time-consuming methodology. In order to quickly detect and classify the skin tumors, the 2D FAA was introduced in this paper. Twenty OCT images per type of skin tumors were randomly chosen from the database. The 2D FAA as well as the 2D DBCM was used to calculate the 2D FD. The FD calculated by using the 2D FAA and the statistical analysis between study groups were showed in **Table 1**. The FD that was obtained by employing the 2D DBCM and the statistical analysis between study groups were showed in **Table 2**. The averaged time for extracting the FD by using the two methodologies was showed in **Table 3**. The results in **Table 1** indicated that the Fourier FD of the basal cell carcinomas is significantly smaller than FD of melanomas. Compared to the FD value of melanomas, the Fourier FD of the basal cell carcinomas has a 2.79% decrease. The results also indicated that the Fourier FD of the benign melanocytic nevi is significantly smaller than FD of melanomas. Compared to the FD value of melanomas, the Fourier FD of the benign melanocytic nevi has a 2.69% decrease. The results in **Table 2** indicated that the FD of the basal cell carcinomas by using the 2D DBCM is significantly smaller than the FD of melanomas. Compared to the melanomas, the DBCM FD of the basal cell carcinomas has a 1.76% decrease. Compared to the melanomas, the DBCM FD of the benign melanocytic nevi showed the same tread. Specifically, the FD (calculated by using the 2D DBCM) of the benign melanocytic nevi decreased 1.38% as compared to the melanomas. In order to compare the computational time between the two methods, we run the two MATLAB codes (ver. R2007b) in the same laptop (i5-4210 CPU, 8GB RAM). In **Table 3**, the computational time was shorter by 91.71% for FAA than 2D DBCM.

Our results showed that the melanomas had a larger FD than the basal cell carcinomas and the benign melanocytic nevi when both of the two methodologies were utilized in the calculations. As the FD is used to express the abnormality of the biological tissue, our results suggested that the melanomas had more irregularity than the basal cell carcinomas and the benign melanocytic nevi. Melanomas feature heavily disorganized vessels with chaotic branching, which might be the explanation for that finding. These specific results indicated that both the Fourier FD and the differential box counting dimension could be used as an indicator to differentiate the melanomas from the basal cell carcinomas and the benign melanocytic nevi. It is worth noting that the Fourier FD is bigger than the differential box counting dimension in our calculations. The Fourier FD was calculated in the frequency domain, while the differential box counting dimension was calculated in the spatial domain. One possible reason to explain the difference is due to the undercount of the number of the boxes in the 2D DBCM which resulted in a small differential box counting dimension in the calculations. Moreover, our results also

Fractal analysis	Melanomas	Basal cell carcinomas	Nevi
FD	2.836 ± 0.031	2.757 ± 0.023[b]	2.760 ± 0.045[b]

[b]$p < 0:001$ (ANOVA followed by Newman-Keuls post hoc analysis) between melanomas and benign melanocytic nevi (see nevi column) and between melanomas and basal cell carcinomas (see basal column)

Table 1.
Distribution of FD (mean ± SD) values calculated by performing the FAA.

Fractal analysis	Melanomas	Basal cell carcinomas	Nevi
FD	2.388 ± 0.011	2.346 ± 0.013[b]	2.355 ± 0.008[b]

[b] $p < 0.001$ *(ANOVA followed by Newman-Keuls post hoc analysis) between melanomas and benign melanocytic nevi (see nevi column) and between melanomas and basal cell carcinomas (see basal column)*

Table 2.
Distribution of FD (mean ± SD) values calculated by using the DBCM.

	Fourier[1]	DBC[2]
Time(s)	0.088 ± 0.003	1.059 ± 0.020

[1]*Fourier: the 2D FAA*
[2]*DBC: the 2D DBCM*

Table 3.
Comparison of the computational time for calculating the FD by using the two methods.

showed that the differences of the Fourier FDs between the melanomas and the basal cell carcinomas are bigger than the differences of the differential box counting dimension, which could lead to a conclusion that the 2D Fourier FD could be better to classify the melanomas from the basal cell carcinomas. Our results also showed that the computational time for calculating 2D Fourier FD is much less than the computational time for calculating the 2D differential box counting dimension. This particular result suggested that the 2D FAA is more efficient to differentiate the skin tumors than the 2D DBCM.

There are several potential shortcomings of our study. The custom-built SD-OCT technology has some limitations as compared to the more pioneering OCT technology. In addition, current OCT devices include different algorithms and methodologies for the removal of the speckle noise. Therefore, data analysis is influenced by special assumptions and technological specifications that are in place for each individual OCT device. Another limitation is that only 20 scans were randomly selected for each type of skin tumors. Thus, more scans would be beneficial for extracting the more accurate FD and find the diagnostic parameter to differentiate the skin tumors.

4. Conclusion

In summary, we have described an efficient approach to calculate the 2D FD form OCT images for classifying the basal cell carcinomas, melanomas, and benign melanocytic nevi in this paper. The preliminary results presented have indicated that the 2D FAA is more efficient for extracting the FD than the 2D DBCM. Particularly, the change in the fractal dimension may reflect the pathological metabolic changes in melanomas. More research studies are needed to determine the accuracy, repeatability, and full capability of this methodology with more OCT images.

Acknowledgements

This research was supported in part by the research grant D2016009 from the Ningbo University of Technology of China and the research grant nos. 2017A610239, 2018A610249, and 2018A610362 from the Ningbo Natural Science Foundation.

Author details

Wei Gao[1], Bingjiang Lin[2*], Valery P. Zakharov[3] and Oleg O. Myakinin[3]

1 School of Safety Engineering, Ningbo University of Technology, Ningbo, China

2 Ningbo First Hospital, Ningbo, China

3 Department of Laser and Biotechnical Systems, Samara National Research University, Samara, Russian Federation

*Address all correspondence to: bingjianglin@foxmail.com

IntechOpen

References

[1] Huang D, Swanson EA, Lin CP, Schuman JS, Stinson WG, Chang W, et al. Optical coherence tomography. Science. 1991;**254**:1178-1181. DOI: 10.1126/science.1957169

[2] Fercher AF, Hitzenberger CK, Drexler W, Kamp G, Sattmann H. *In vivo* optical coherence tomography. American Journal of Ophthalmology. 1993;**116**(1):113-114. DOI: 10.1016/S0002-9394(14)71762-3

[3] Kim KH, Pierce MC, Maguluri G, Park BH, Yoon SJ, Lydon M, et al. *In vivo* imaging of human burn injuries with polarization-sensitive optical coherence tomography. Journal of Biomedical Optics. 2012;**17**(6):066012. DOI: 10.1117/1.JBO.17.6.066012

[4] Mogensen M, Thrane L, Jorgensen TM, Andersen PE, Jemec GB. OCT imaging of skin cancer and other dermatological diseases. Journal of Biophotonics. 2009;**2**(6-7):442-451. DOI: 10.1002/jbio.200910020

[5] Barui A, Banerjee P, Patra R, Das RK, Dutta PK, Chatterjee J. Swept-source optical coherence tomography of lower limb wound healing with histopathological correlation. Journal of Biomedical Optics. 2011;**16**(2):026010. DOI: 10.1117/1.3535593

[6] Mogensen M, Nurnberg BM, Thrane L, Jorgensen TM, Andersen PE, Jemec GB. How histological features of basal cell carcinomas influence image quality in optical coherence tomography. Journal of Biophotonics. 2011;**4**(7-8):544-551. DOI: 10.1002/jbio.201100006

[7] Gan Y, Tsay D, Amir SB, Marboe CC, Hendon CP. Automated classification of optical coherence tomography images of human atrial tissue. Journal of Biomedical Optics. 2016;**21**(10):101407. DOI: 10.1117/1.jbo.21.10.101407

[8] Marvdashti T, Duan L, Ransohoff KJ, Aasi SZ, Tang JY, Ellerbee AK. Towards automated detection of basal cell carcinoma from polarization sensitive optical coherence tomography images of human skin. In: Conference on Lasers and Electro-Optics Europe—Technical Digest 2015; Cleo; 7184045. DOI: 10.1364/CLEO_SI.2015.STh3K.3

[9] Lingley-Papadopoulos CA, Loew MH, Manyak MJ. Computer recognition of cancer in the urinary bladder using optical coherence tomography and texture analysis. Journal of Biomedical Optics. 2008;**13**(2):024003. DOI: 10.1117/1.2904987

[10] Gambichler T, Schmid-Wendtner MH, Plura I, Kampilafkos P, Stücker M, Berking C, et al. A multicentre pilot study investigating high-definition optical coherence tomography in the differentiation of cutaneous melanoma and melanocytic nevi. Journal of the European Academy of Dermatology and Venereology. 2015;**29**(3):537-541. DOI: 10.1111/jdv.12621

[11] Wahrlich C, Alawi SA, Batz S, Fluhr JW, Lademann J, Ulrich M. Assessment of a scoring system for basal cell carcinoma with multi-beam optical coherence tomography. Journal of the European Academy of Dermatology and Venereology. 2015;**29**(8):1562-1569. DOI: 10.1111/jdv.12935

[12] Ashok PC, Praveen BB, Bellini N, Riches A, Dholakia K, Herrington CS. Multi-modal approach using Raman spectroscopy and optical coherence tomography for the discrimination of colonic adenocarcinoma from normal colon. Biomedical Optics Express. 2013;**4**(10):002179. DOI: 10.1364/BOE.4.002179

[13] Bhattacharjee M, Ashok PC, Rao KD, Majumder SK, Verma Y,

Gupta PK. Binary tissue classification studies on resected human breast tissues using optical coherence tomography images. Journal of Innovative Optical Health Sciences. 2011;**4**(1):59-66. DOI: 10.1142/S1793545811001083

[14] Mandelbrog BB. How long is the coast of Britian? Statistical self-similarity and fractal dimension. Science. 1967;**156**:636-638. DOI: 10.1126/science.156.3775.636

[15] Hussain RJ, Deviha VS, Rengarajan P. Analysing the invasiveness of skin cancer using fractals. International Journal of Engineering Research and Applications. 2012;**2**:2068-2075

[16] Karimi T, Farshchi SMR. Skin cancer expert system using fractal dimension. Research Journal of Pure Algebra. 2012;**2**:88-97

[17] Gao W, Zakharov VP, Myakinin OO, Bratchenko IA, Artemyev DN, Kornilin DV. Medical images classification for skin cancer using quantitative image features with optical coherence tomography. Journal of Innovative Optical Health Sciences. 2016;**9**(2):1650003. DOI: 10.1142/S1793545816500036

[18] Salinas HM, Fernandez DC. Comparison of PDE-based nonlinear diffusion approaches for image enhancement and denoising in optical coherence tomography. IEEE Transactions on Medical Imaging. 2007;**26**:761-771. DOI: 10.1109/TMI.2006.887375

[19] Puvanathasan P, Bizheva K. Interval type-II fuzzy anisotropic diffusion algorithm for speckle noise reduction in optical coherence tomography images. Optical Express. 2009;**17**:733-746. DOI: 10.1364/OE.17.000733

[20] Long M, Peng F. A box-counting method with adaptable box height for measuring the fractal feature of images. Radioengineering. 2013;**22**:208-213

[21] Ahammer H. Higuchi dimension of digital images. PLoS ONE. 2011;**6**:e24796. DOI: 10.1371/journal.pone.0024796

[22] Sarkar N, Chaudhuri BB. An efficient approach to estimate fractal dimension of textural images. Pattern Recognition. 1992;**25**:1035-1041. DOI: 10.1016/0031-3203(92)90066-r

www.ingramcontent.com/pod-product-compliance
Lightning Source LLC
Chambersburg PA
CBHW081233190326
41458CB00016B/5766